613.7

613.7

D0305741

THE COMPLETE ILLUSTRATED GUIDE TO

YOGA

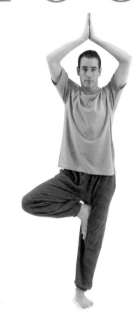

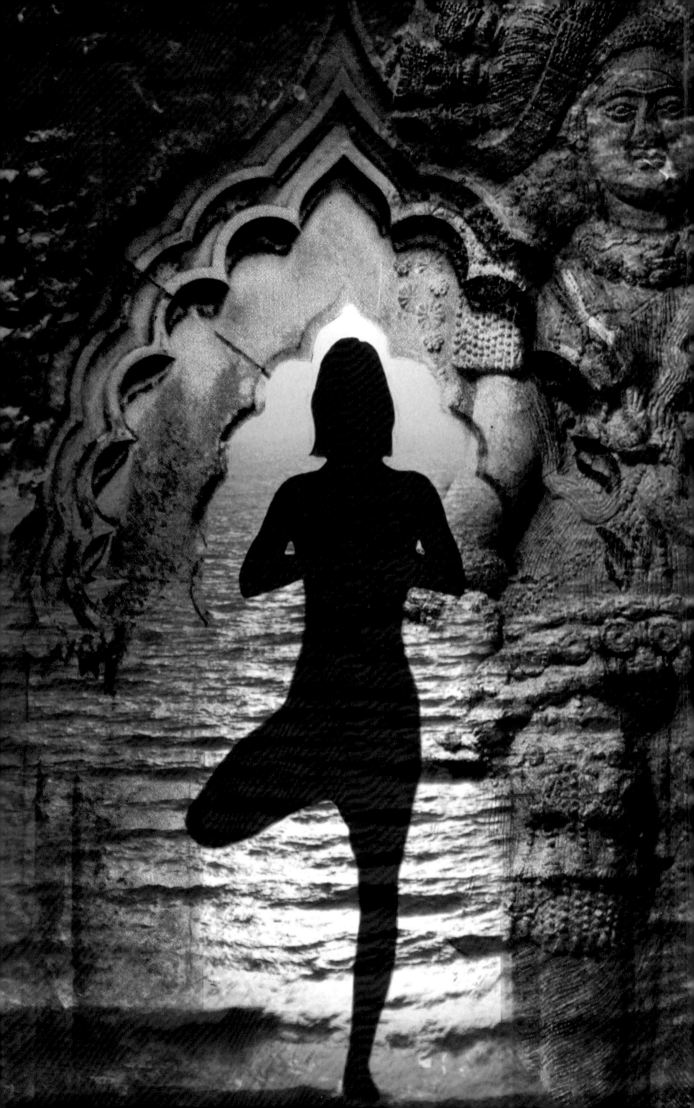

THE COMPLETE ILLUSTRATED GUIDE TO
YOGA

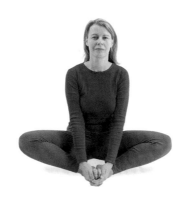

A practical approach to achieving optimum health for mind, body, and spirit

HOWARD KENT

ELEMENT

Shaftesbury, Dorset • Boston, Massachusetts • Melbourne, Victoria

© Element Books Limited 1999

First published in Great Britain in 1999 by
ELEMENT BOOKS LIMITED
Shaftesbury, Dorset SP7 8BP

Published in the USA in 1999 by
ELEMENT BOOKS INC
160 North Washington Street, Boston MA 02114

Published in Australia in 1999 by
ELEMENT BOOKS LIMITED
and distributed by Penguin Australia Ltd
487 Maroondah Highway, Ringwood, Victoria 3134

Note from the Publisher
Any information given in this book is not intended to be taken
as a replacement for medical advice. Any person with a condition requiring
medical attention should consult a qualified practitioner or therapist.

Designed and created for Element Books with
THE BRIDGEWATER BOOK COMPANY LIMITED

ELEMENT BOOKS LIMITED
Editorial Director: SUE HOOK
Managing Editor: MIRANDA SPICER
Senior Commissioning Editor: CARO NESS
Project Editor: FINNY FOX-DAVIES
Group Production Director: CLARE ARMSTRONG
Production Manager: STEPHANIE RAGGETT
Production Controller: FIONA HARRISON

THE BRIDGEWATER BOOK COMPANY
Art Director: TERRY JEAVONS
Editorial Director: FIONA BIGGS
Designer: SARAH HOWERD
Page Make-up: PAUL MESSAM AND SARA KIDD
Managing Editor: ANNE TOWNLEY
Picture research: VANESSA FLETCHER
Illustrator: MIKE COURTNEY
Three-dimensional models: MARK JAMIESON
Studio Photography: MIKE HEMSLEY AT WALTER GARDINER STUDIOS

Printed and bound in Great Britain by
Butler & Tanner

Library of Congress Cataloging in Publication
data available

ISBN 1 86204 456 2 Hardback
ISBN 1 86204 455 4 Paperback

Contents

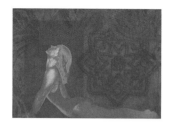

Part Six
The Positions

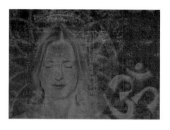

Part Seven
Breathing Techniques

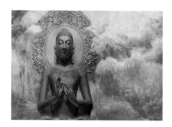

Part Eight
Meditation

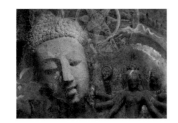

Part Nine
Philosophy of Yoga

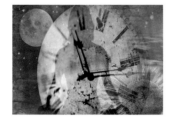

Part Ten
Yoga in Daily Life

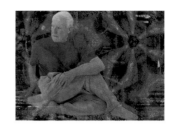

Part Eleven
Yoga for Special Needs

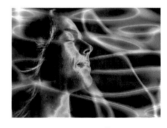

Part Twelve
Yoga and Healing

How to Use this Book

The *Complete Illustrated Guide to Yoga* is a comprehensive introduction to an ancient practice that is becoming more and more popular in response to the pressures of modern life. Most people think of yoga as a kind of advanced Eastern exercise program; in fact yoga is a lifestyle that embraces mind, body, and spirit. Through meditation, control of breathing, and correct posture, yoga seeks to release the life force (called prana by the yoga sages) so that it flows naturally through every part of our being.

This book is divided into 12 parts. **Parts 1 and 2** look at the history and origins of yoga, and the benefits it can bring. **Parts 3 and 4** show how yoga works in harmony with the body's natural design. In **Parts 5, 6, and 7**, the physical exercises, called asanas, are introduced, together with other exercises to encourage breathing and circulation. **Parts 8 and 9** consider the meditative and spiritual aspects of yoga. The final section of the book, **Parts 10, 11, and 12**, relates what has been presented earlier to our daily lives, including yoga for special needs and yoga for healing.

Right: The central section of the book gives detailed descriptions of the different exercises that have been developed over the ages to stimulate the flow of prana through the body. There is information on how to begin the practice of yoga, and how to create a program that suits your own needs.

Planning a Yoga Program

In some ways the idea of planning a yoga program runs agai behind yoga practice. Everyone's physiology and psychology a the aim of yoga is to learn to listen to the body's own needs a wants to do. However, while some people work effectively in way, others need to follow a set program, especially when the

Before planning their program, all students should sit and think carefully about why they want to take up yoga and what they want to achieve. It is important to be realistic from the start: however enthusiastically you practice, yoga may never give you a more shapely body or make you lose weight. Focus on the idea that the main objective of yoga is to bring inner peace and harmony (see pages 18–19).

Yoga can fit very comfortably into different lifestyles. There is no ideal time of day to practice – yogis traditionally practice asanas for most of the day. Individual lifestyle dictates the time of day the sessions take place. There is only one rule: to be effective, practice must be regular – once a week at least, preferably three or four times a week, ideally once a day. There is no set duration for a class. The planner illustrated opposite allocates time for a 90-minute class, since 90 minutes is an optimum timespan for the human body (see pages 26–27), but it is possible to benefit from daily sessions lasting for 20–30 minutes each, or sessions that vary in duration from day to day and increase over time.

There are certain elements that every yoga program needs. Each session should begin with a few stretches and a moment of stillness, plus a few minutes of relaxation through breathing. Time working on the asanas needs to be punctuated by brief relaxation breaks. The session should end with breathing practice and several minutes of full relaxation.

Many yoga manuals suggest that the asanas should be practiced in a certain order based on the progressive exercising of different parts of the body. These considerations are not important, however. The asanas in this book may b practiced in almost any orde with the one proviso that is essential to observe principle of balance and co terbalance – a forward b ward bend, and so on (see p

At first, students often f greater flexibility in the spin asanas affecting other parts want to work on a stiff nec arms. It is perfectly possible one session and the hands another, and to plan short se ance or breathing. What is i yoga program is to keep the whole picture in mind se that no part of the body i ignored.

Making progress means that the program will nee to be replanned at interval Beginners may prefer to co centrate on exercise a breathing at the beginning a only try meditation and visu ization (see pages 126–29) w they feel more confident.

Follow a backward bend with one that flexes the spine in the opposite direction.

A forward bend counteracts the effect of a backward be

60

MAIN TEXT EXPLAINS
HOW YOGA BENEFITS
MIND AND BODY

X-RAY PHOTOGRAPHY
HIGHLIGHTS SPECIFIC BODY
SYSTEMS THAT YOGA ADDRESSES

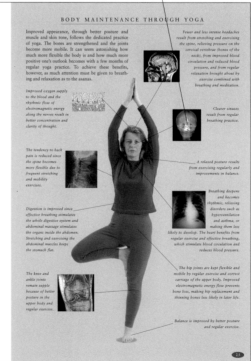

Benefits of Yoga

The body is an energy system with close interplay between breathing, heart beat, and brain function. Yoga provides a maintenance service for that system. Rightly described as "the heart of healing," yoga also provides a harmonizing process that leaves no part of the body untouched.

Working from the premise that "Life is breath, breath is life," yoga places great emphasis on making the breathing deep, rhythmic, and effective. Respiration, the thinking goes, is not just a matter of exchanging gases, it is also the body's pumping system. The diaphragm (the large muscle that stretches across the body between the chest and the abdomen) forms a cone during inhalation, which acts as the piston of body energy. To function effectively it depends upon the movement of the lower ribs, and these depend upon posture and natural breathing to work properly themselves.

Respiration is the source of oxygen and other gases that fuel the body. They penetrate the lung tissues to dissolve in the blood, and they are pumped along with other nutrients through tiny capillaries to nourish the extremities of the body, and through major arteries to the great organs, such as the brain. To work effectively the brain requires not only effective oxygenation but also a rhythmic flow of electromagnetic energy, generated by the heart and transported by the nerves. Without these, essential thoughts and messages will be muddled and negative, and the body will suffer from tiredness and incapacity.

Yoga asanas and yogic breathing stimulate the nervous system, clearing the body's electromagnetic energy pathways to and from the brain. This is one channel through which breathing affects outlook. Poor breathing may not always be the cause of low spirits, but shallow or irregular breathing invariably accompany attacks of depression and other mood swings and disorders. The heart, like the breath, responds to the mind's perceptions of life.

Electrocardiograms show the damage caused by habitually negative thoughts, and conversely the healing process that may be brought about by more positive ones.

Even the bony skeleton of the body is affected by the mental and physical harmony that yoga can bring about. Bone, like other tissue, is constantly renewing itself, and the body's electromagnetic energy plays a central part in this renewal, so yoga helps maintain bone density. The joints require balanced use if they are to work well. The interplay between mental calmness, free flow of the breath, and harmonized movement, provided by yoga, helps to maintain this balance.

Because of its emphasis on balanced stretching and exercise, yoga can be used to prevent and ease many painful conditions caused by the overuse of joints and limbs, from hamstring and other sports injuries to a frozen shoulder. It can also provide short-term remedies for complaints caused by stress, including tension headaches and hyperventilation (fast, shallow breathing).

Yoga encourages heart and brain to function freely, unhampered by stress. Although it can take long and regular practice to restore some of the damage caused by years of neglect, beginners can take heart from the knowledge that improvement can be seen in many aspects of body function and mental outlook after just a few sessions. In the long term, however, yoga brings about emotional control, resulting in a peaceful state of mind and a calm lifestyle, and more effective functioning of every part of the body.

The tree posture is one of many asanas that improve balance and coordination.

BODY MAINTENANCE THROUGH YOGA

Improved appearance, through better posture and muscle and skin tone, follows the dedicated practice of yoga. The bones are strengthened and the joints become more mobile. It can seem astonishing how much more flexible the body is and how much more positive one's outlook becomes with a few months of regular yoga practice. To achieve these benefits, however, as much attention must be given to breathing and relaxation as to the asanas.

Improved oxygen supply to the blood and the rhythmic flow of electromagnetic energy along the nerves result in better concentration and clarity of thought.

The tendency to back pain is reduced since the spine becomes more flexible due to frequent stretching and mobility exercises.

Digestion is improved since effective breathing stimulates the whole digestive system and abdominal massage stimulates the organs inside the abdomen. Stretching and exercising the abdominal muscles keep the stomach flat.

The knee and ankle joints remain supple because of better posture in the upper body and regular exercise.

Fewer and less intense headaches result from stretching and exercising the spine, relieving pressure on the cervical vertebrae (bones of the neck), from improved blood circulation and reduced blood pressure, and from regular relaxation brought about by exercise combined with breathing and meditation.

Clearer sinuses result from regular breathing practice.

A relaxed posture results from exercising regularly and improvements in balance.

Breathing deepens and becomes rhythmic, relieving disorders such as hyperventilation and asthma, or making them less likely to develop. The heart benefits from regular exercise and effective breathing, which stimulate blood circulation and reduces blood pressure.

The hip joints are kept flexible and mobile by regular exercise and correct carriage of the upper body. Improved electromagnetic energy flow prevents bone loss, making hip replacement and thinning bones less likely in later life.

Balance is improved by better posture and regular exercise.

24

25

Left: The first part of the book explores the anatomical basis of yoga practice, looking at the ways in which yoga works to improve circulation, develop good posture, and most importantly encourage and sustain correct breathing.

GUIDANCE IS GIVEN ON HOW TO DEVELOP A PROGRAM OF ASANAS

CLEAR STEP-BY-STEP PHOTOGRAPHS WITH CAPTIONS SHOW HOW TO PERFORM EACH ASANA

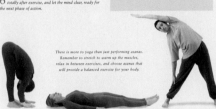

ESSENTIAL ELEMENTS OF A PROGRAM

Objective: To improve the quality of my life.

Although yoga is partly physical, the exercise is merely a means to attain the mental calm needed for meditation. Beware of the mindset that idealizes physical perfection. In yoga the body does not always "improve" from an aesthetic point of view. But if you allow yoga to bring you inner happiness you may find your appearance changes.

1 Warm-up stretches – 10 minutes: These relax the muscles and joints, warm the body, and speed the circulation ready for practice. Stretching banishes the stresses and excitements of the day, clears the mind, and focuses on the yoga session.

2 Relaxation – 1 minute: Always rest the muscles and joints for a short time after using them. Allow the mind to clear and focus on the next phase of action.

3 Breathing – 10 minutes: This cools off the body after vigorous exercise, slows the heartbeat, and induces greater flexibility. Breathing calms the thoughts, sharpens receptivity, and provides a pause for listening to the body and gauging what it wants.

4 Asanas sequence – 50 minutes: The sequence improves mobility, flexibility, and muscle control. It trains the mind in concentration and control of thoughts and emotions.

5 Breath Control – 10 minutes: This energizes the body's neuro-electrical system and generates a state of calm.

6 Full relaxation – 10 minutes: Allow the body to rest totally after exercise, and let the mind clear, ready for the next phase of action.

SUGGESTED ASANA SEQUENCE	
ACTION	TIME
Half lotus	5 minutes
Cat and Dog	10 minutes
Pause to rest	1 minute
Spinal twist	10 minutes
Pause to rest	1 minute
Triangle and reverse triangle	5 minutes
Pause to rest	1 minute
Bow	5 minutes
Boat	5 minutes
Pause to rest	1 minute
Half candle	5 minutes

There is more to yoga than just performing asanas. Remember to stretch to warm up the muscles, relax in between exercises, and choose asanas that will provide a balanced exercise for your body.

Stretching the Spine

The vertebrae – the bones, some fused, others that make up the spine – work together to give the movement. Slipped disks and other problems occur in the way it should be. Perhaps as much as 80 pain is due to poor posture, and so is preventable.

keep the spine flexible will never experience that problem. The same is true of other back complaints – slipped disks are the culminating disaster in a series of spinal injuries which began, most often, with bad posture that was never corrected. The stretches illustrated on the next few pages are the first steps in encouraging the spine's natural flexibility to reassert itself.

POSTERIOR STRETCH

is designed to counter the compressing action on the spine. Do not try to force the spine to further than it can easily go. Just follow the movements and concentrate on the breathing. any stiffness will ease and your back will begin to bend more easily.

1 Sit on the floor with your legs in front of you. Your feet should be a hand's breadth apart and pointing upward. Sit with your spine and head erect and your hands resting on the floor at your sides. Breathe slowly out, then inhale while lifting your arms right above your head and raising your trunk, stretching all the muscles of the back. Keep the backs of your legs on the floor.

2 Breathing out, and with your back still lifted and your arms extended slowly, stretch forward slowly. Keep the backs of your legs on the floor. Concentrate your thoughts on stretching forward.

3 As the out-breath ends, lower your arms to grasp your legs as far down as you can reach – the calves, the ankles, the toes. Drop your head and relax for at least half a minute, breathing gently while continuing to stretch.

COBRA

This bend, which imitates the rearing movement of a cobra, stretches the front of the body and counterbalances the posterior stretch.

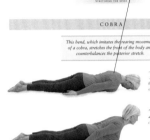

1 Lie face down, with your forehead resting on the mat and your arms by your sides, palms upward. Breathe out slowly.

2 Breathe in, lifting first your head, then your neck, shoulders, and chest from the mat.

3 As soon as you feel you have lifted your head as far as you can, or if your back is weak or has been injured, move your arms forward so that you rest on your forearms, palms down.

4 On an in-breath, continue to lift the upper body while keeping your hips and legs on the floor. When you feel able, straighten your arms and rest your weight on the palms of your hands. Close your eyes and breathe slowly for at least half a minute. Then, breathing out, slowly lower the upper body and move your arms back to your sides, until you are lying as you were in step 1. Relax.

5 Repeat steps 1–4 at each daily practice. Concentrate on your breathing and on stretching a little further back each time. As your spine becomes more flexible you will find you move your hands gradually closer to your body.

INTRODUCTORY PANELS DESCRIBE THE PURPOSE OF EACH ASANA

Dealing with Other People

The great spiritual teachings have much in common, most notably their rules of behavior. All have urged us to treat others as we would have them treat us. These similarities come as no surprise to followers of yoga, who believe that the universe and its inhabitants are subject to a network of laws governing thought and action. People may choose whether to obey them, but if they do not, they will not feel happy and may not remain healthy.

Almost everyone can remember disregarding the rule, "Do as you would be done by," with disastrous effects on peace of mind. There are five yamas as guidelines for our behavior toward other people. There are five principal yamas, but some texts list up to ten. Some may be read as examples, rather than taken literally. Ksama, for instance, exhorts everyone to accept abuse or apparent ill treatment quietly and not to respond in kind, like Christ turning the other cheek. It may be interpreted in a modern sense as good advice on refusing to let people irritate you.

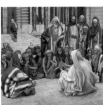

Faithfulness in sexual relationships is one aspect of right living.

Failing to obey these 2,000-year-old principles will, even now, do nobody any good. The injunction not to get involved in violence, for example, stems from understanding that thought vibrations that cause violent action only result in more violence, harming the attacker and the victim. In yoga, the end never justifies violent means, even if the goal is to overthrow a tyrant.

Yoga does not only set rules, it provides workable techniques for training oneself to follow them. It teaches mind and body how to calm ruffled emotions and stifle society's conditioning to reply in kind, so that the senses remain under the will's command in all circumstances. Medical research into stress during the 20th century has demonstrated the effectiveness of the yoga approach.

THE FIVE YAMAS

ONE
To refrain from violence, in thought, word, or deed
The elimination of all violence from our relationships with others is the first yama, called ahimsa. This means never blaming other people for things that happen; never speaking harsh words to another; never hurting any person by thought, speech, or action; and never killing anyone. Since World War II it has become almost acceptable for a head of state to take military action to prevent worse violence by an enemy state. Yet the principle of ahimsa was the one adopted by Mahatma Gandhi when he urged that perceived wrongs should never be opposed by the further wrong of violence.

TWO
To refrain from stealing
Asteya means never taking anything that belongs to others. It extends beyond the theft of objects to include possessions in the widest sense. Wrongfully appropriating thoughts and ideas is theft, too. In modern society a lot of stealing goes on under the guise of being alert and competitive in a hard commercial world.

THREE
To avoid covetousness
Yoga teachings do not demand a vow of poverty, but they insist that possessiveness should be avoided. True peace of mind does not come from collecting material objects. If we make a point of holding on to them we create harmful inhibitions in ourselves and in those with whom we are in contact.

FOUR
To speak the truth
The sage Vyasa defined truth as follows: "that which is beneficial to beings, spoken justly, and the agreeable is also said to be true." In other words, there is a tendency for us to tell half-truths in order to save ourselves embarrassment – or to gain some benefit or even to wound. Satya means always speaking the truth. In the end it will bring the greatest benefit.

FIVE
To refrain from sexual depravity
The yamas were once generally expounded to members of religious groups, who had taken vows to remain celibate. For others, brahmacharya may be interpreted as "love, not lust, and faithfulness in marriage." Strict social rules governing normal sexual behavior may not be as relevant as they once were, yet this yama is still necessary. The effects of the actions of those who give way to depraved lust cause indescribable misery to children forced into prostitution in countries all over the world.

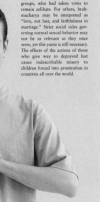

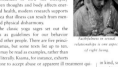

Mahatma Gandhi inspired millions with his refusal to use violence in his struggle for Indian independence.

Jesus Christ preached nonviolence as a way of life, turning the other cheek as the answer to hostility.

Left: *The final section of the book looks at the ways in which the yoga lifestyle reaches into every aspect of our daily lives, from the food we eat to the demands of other people and the problems of illness or psychological distress.*

Introduction

················

In the 19th century a handful of Western scholars became interested in Eastern cultures and first introduced yoga to the West. At first, this ancient discipline was derided. It nonetheless caught on because those who tried it found that it worked. British administrators posted to India, who became interested in its history and culture, became yoga's first teachers.

The 20th century saw the appearance of many new yoga teachers in the West, among them Richard Hittleman, who learned yoga from an Asian servant at home in the US. In the 1960s he became the first teacher of yoga to appear on television. I arranged for Hittleman to come to Britain in 1970 to make a television series which was screened in 20 countries. Michael Volin, a Russian born in 1915 in China, who studied in India and Tibet, became the father of the yoga movement in Australia. Britain's first yoga organization, the British Wheel of Yoga, was started in the 1960s by the army officer Wilfred Clarke, who became interested in yoga during World War I.

Indian yogis soon began to teach in the West. One of the best known is B.K.S. Iyengar, who after World War II opened schools in Britain and the US. One of his earliest students was the world-famous violinist Yehudi Menuhin, who asked the teacher for help in restoring movement to a frozen shoulder. A program of gentle exercise and relaxation restored the flow of energy to the joint, and the violinist sent Iyengar a wristwatch inscribed, "To my best violin teacher."

The growth in popularity of yoga in the West took place at the same time as a remarkable phenomenon of mind and body was being researched, now called stress. As the pace of life quickened and pressures mounted, feelings of mental unease were often accompanied by symptoms of physical illness. These are now known to be the result of harmful psychophysical effects. Increasingly, the role of yoga as an effective means of mitigating chronic pain, illness, and disability is being recognized, with a small but growing number of research papers now available.

Perhaps of greater benefit is the effectiveness of yoga in helping to prevent ill health. Routine exhortations not to smoke, drink in excess, or take drugs, and recommendations to exercise regularly, certainly have value, but they do not necessarily bring peace of mind. This is where yoga comes into its own. Many people who have managed to resolve a crisis successfully now say, "I don't know how I would have coped if it hadn't been for yoga."

This book is for everyone who is considering taking up yoga, and for those who have already

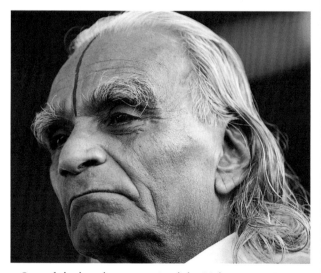

One of the best-known yogis of the 20th century, B.K.S. Iyengar has established his own style of yoga.

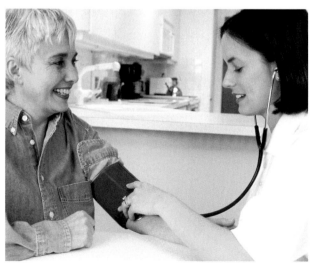

Yoga provides a gentle cure for modern complaints such as high blood pressure.

walked a short way along its path. Its approach is simple: the various exercises and asanas (postures) illustrated and described have been chosen from among the many possible variations because they are fundamental and useful.

The purpose is not just to teach the basics of yoga, but to show that yoga is more than simply a set of physical exercises. The asanas without their mental and spiritual background are not really yoga.

This is a book for children, young adults, the middle-aged, and the elderly, because yoga is a pursuit that should last a lifetime. It is not just for the fit. The Yoga for Health Foundation which I began in 1976 in England now has representatives in 23 countries. Many of their students are sick, convalescent, or disabled, and this book is also for them and people like them the world over.

Yoga is a holistic therapy which has a spiritual as well as a physical aspect.

CAUTION

Yoga stretches and asanas should always be practiced gently, with the correct breathing. Attempting unfamiliar asanas without first preparing the muscles and tendons by stretching and breathing, trying to do too much too quickly, and forcing the body into unfamiliar positions will cause damage. The back is especially vulnerable. If the spine is stiff it must be eased very gently into stretches and twists. Trying to maintain an erect posture is the best exercise for it at first. Forcing it to bend can damage it permanently.

Students learning yoga alone need to be particularly cautious and to progress slowly. Interpret pain as a warning sign and stop immediately it occurs. Try the posture a day later and the pain may not recur.

Anyone who has a medical condition should ask for expert advice before beginning yoga. It is sensible to consult a physician and ask for a note identifying the condition to show to the yoga teacher. For a second opinion about any problem that occurs in a yoga class it may be possible to check with a recognized and reputable non-commercial yoga organization, or even a therapist in a different discipline, such as chiropractic, osteopathy, or naturopathy.

CHECK LIST

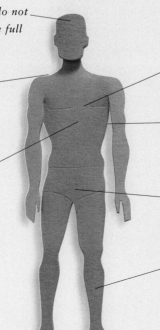

Migraines: *do not attempt the full candle.*

Back: *if you have back pain do not attempt the boat asana or the shoulder stands, which strain the back.*

Chest: *if you have asthma, bronchitis, emphysema, or other serious chest complaints do not attempt the special breathing techniques or the uddiyana bandha movement (see pages 106-7).*

Heart problems and high blood pressure: *do not do any inverted postures.*

Osteoporosis: *stretch and exercise the back very gently and do not attempt the boat asana or the shoulder stands.*

Hernias of the abdomen, chest, or groin: *do not attempt forward bends.*

Varicose veins: *do not sit in cross-legged positions.*

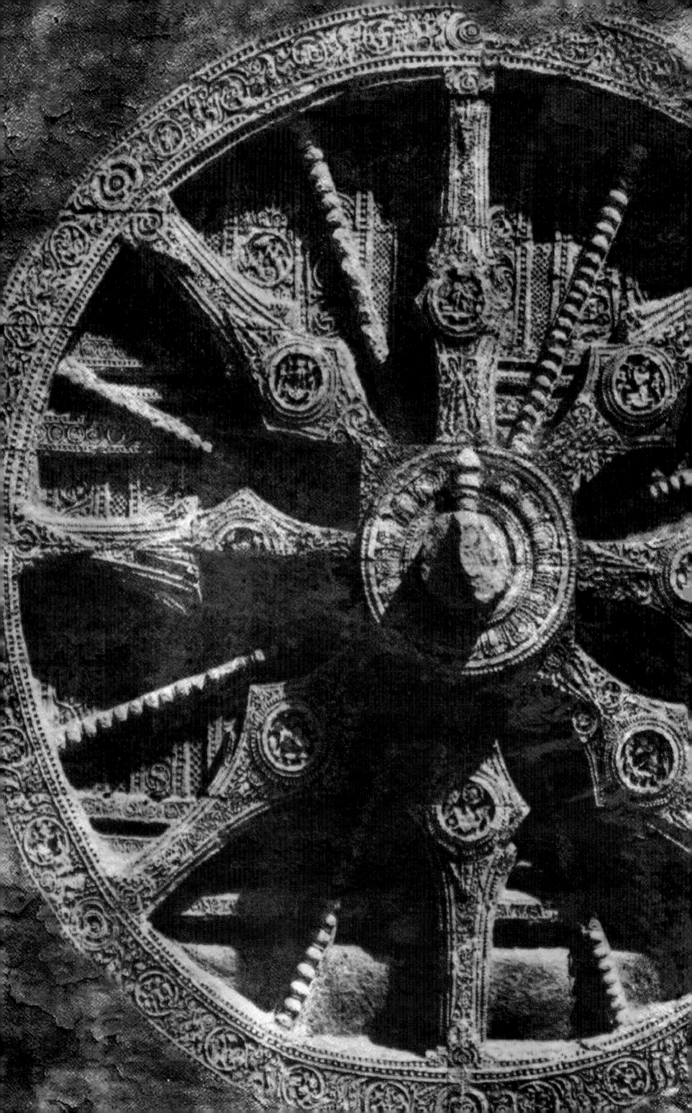

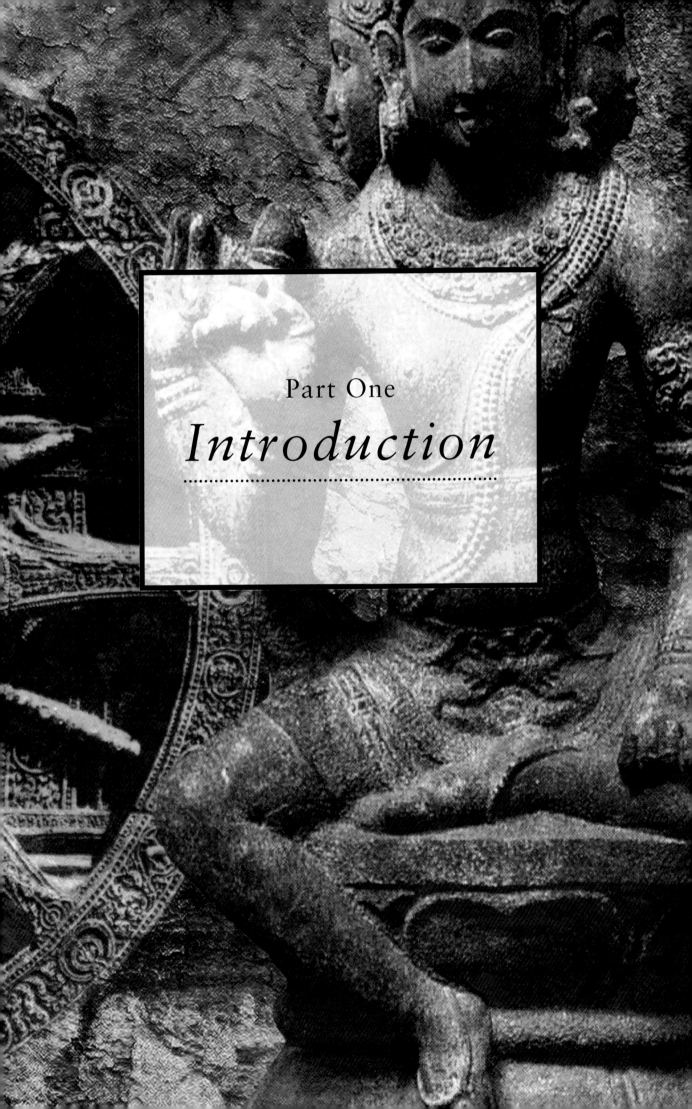

Part One
Introduction

Origins of Yoga

·····································

The ideas and practices that became known as yoga may have arisen among the Aryans, a group of nomadic tribes that originated in south Russia. When they migrated from Persia into India during the second millennium BCE, they may have shared their ideas with the Dravidian-speaking peoples of the subcontinent.

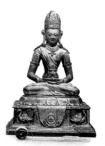

Meditation is central to yoga.

The word "yoga" comes from Sanskrit, the great classical language of ancient India. Its principal meaning is oneness, expressing the belief that the individual is part of the universal whole. (Yoga is often linked with the word "yug," meaning to yoke, but the yoke was a later invention.) Statuettes, official seals, and other artifacts found in archeological sites on the Indian subcontinent show men meditating in the lotus position. What these and other finds suggest is the belief that the understanding of existence could be found by developing the ability to be still, to control the mind, and to sit unmoving for considerable lengths of time.

It is often suggested that yoga is an integral part of Hinduism. But in his *History of Yoga*, Vivian Worthington writes, "Yoga has ... tended all along to be anti-intellectual, even antireligious. To be true to itself it must ever stand close to the spontaneous fount of human creativity." Because yoga developed alongside Hinduism, Buddhism, and Jainism, there are links with all these beliefs, but in the ancient East, yogis associated with groups of independent thinkers, the Sramanas, who were sometimes tolerated but were often hunted down and killed when the Hindu priests

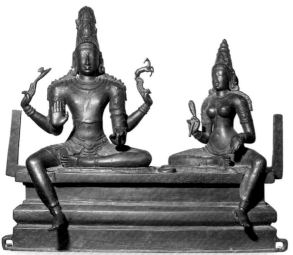

Krishna and Parvati, two divine figures from the Hindu pantheon. Yoga may predate the earliest human religions.

felt their power threatened. Furthermore, early orthodox Hindu beliefs involved sacrificing animals and also, possibly, human beings. Yoga, by contrast, has always been grounded in total respect for life, expressed in the word "ahimsa," which means leading one's life wholly without violence in thought, word, and deed. Vegetarianism has always been central to Indian yoga practices.

Between 200 BCE and 200 CE a remarkable saga, the *Mahabharata* (literally, *Great India*), was compiled, of which one section was entitled the *Bhagavad Gita* (translated as *The Song of God* by Edwin Arnold, former editor of the London *Daily Telegraph*). The *Bhagavad Gita* contains yoga terms and concepts to help the seeker establish how to face one's duty in life. Although it is set on a battlefield, this has been thought by many, including the Indian spiritual leader, Mahatma Ghandi, to be allegorical, showing how the challenges of life should be faced. Humans are enjoined to act dispassionately, "to do the thing that has to be done, because it has to be done and for no other reason." The discipline of yoga, it says, enables its followers to meet this challenge and to move into a state of peace and harmony.

During the 2nd century BCE the teacher Patañjali produced what has become the principal manual of yoga instruction, outlining step by step how to bring the thoughts and mind under control and, from this ultimately to move into the state of ananda, or bliss.

While knowledge and understanding of yoga have advanced remarkably in the West in recent years, many people still equate it with a form of exercise. This is hatha yoga (pronounced "hatta"), the most recent major development of yoga, which originated perhaps a thousand years ago. Those who practice hatha yoga begin by attempting a series of asanas – a Sanskrit word meaning "holding a position." However, hatha yoga did not come into being as a kind of Indian physical jerks but as the consolidation of the different aspects of human life: the body; the flow of energy; the brain, the mind, and the consciousness.

THE SPREAD OF YOGA

Yoga developed on the Indian subcontinent more than 4,000 years ago, from where it was carried by traveling yogis to other Asian countries. As a result of the Muslim invasions of India, which began in 1200 CE, the Sufis, an Islamic sect of freethinking mystics, transmitted it westward to many countries of the Middle East. Interest in the West began in the 1800s when Western scholars translated the ancient Indian texts. This resulted in visits to Britain and the US by swamis (holy men), such as Vivekenanda, who in 1893 attended the World Parliament of Religions in Chicago. During the twentieth century yoga has continued to spread, and today the Yoga for Health Foundation is represented in 24 countries.

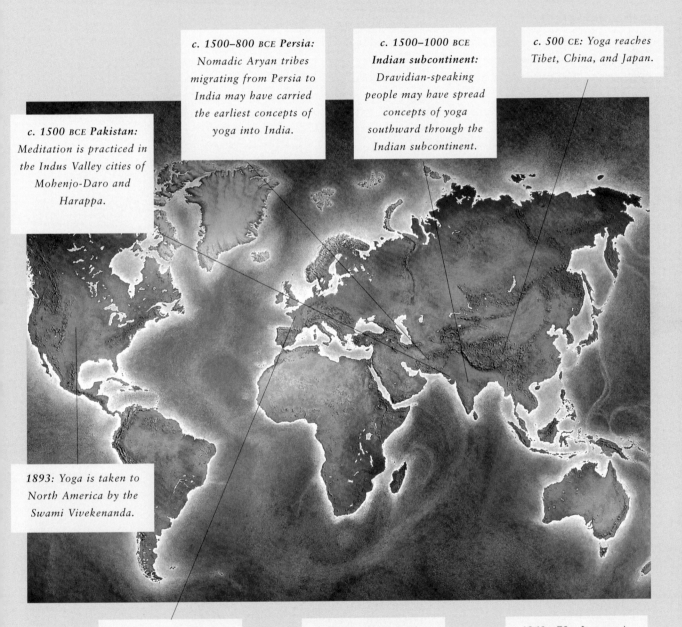

c. 1500–800 BCE Persia: Nomadic Aryan tribes migrating from Persia to India may have carried the earliest concepts of yoga into India.

c. 1500–1000 BCE Indian subcontinent: Dravidian-speaking people may have spread concepts of yoga southward through the Indian subcontinent.

c. 500 CE: Yoga reaches Tibet, China, and Japan.

c. 1500 BCE Pakistan: Meditation is practiced in the Indus Valley cities of Mohenjo-Daro and Harappa.

1893: Yoga is taken to North America by the Swami Vivekenanda.

1800s: Yoga is brought to Europe and Britain by colonial administrators, soldiers, and scholars returning from residence in India.

1900s: Tours and demonstrations by leading yogis, the publication of their works, and the later televising of talks and demonstrations results in the spread of yoga worldwide.

1960s–70s: Interest in Asian ideas and cultures fueled by the advent of less expensive air travel results in an explosion in yoga classes in the West, especially in Britain and North America.

Great Teachers

·····························

Yoga is older than archeology, its historians believe, and its canon incorporates the beliefs, techniques, and practices contributed by generations of anonymous teachers. A very few revered names have survived, only to have been claimed by the major religions of the ancient world as their own great teachers.

Among these can be counted the Buddha because yoga practice has always been central to Buddhism, and enlightenment is still the principal objective of yoga. Another is Mahavira, the founder of modern Jainism, who lived at the turn of the 4th century BCE.

Apart from Patañjali (see pages 14–15), whose teachings have survived in written form as *The Yoga Sutras* (*The Aphorisms of Yoga*), the early sages appear to have been mythical or to have proved to be a complex of different figures. It seems certain, however, that a yogi named Svatmarama lived around the 14th century CE and produced a work called the *Hathapradipika* (*The Compendium of Hatha Yoga*). This outlines the principal hatha asanas – the postures taught in hatha yoga – and makes it clear that these are not only body movements but are also aimed at controlling the mind. In fact, Svatmarama suggests that the physical techniques of yoga are part of the learning process only, and are intended to be discarded as one moves further along the path.

A major figure of the 19th century was Ramakrishna, born into a poor Calcutta family in 1836, who became a Brahman – a Hindu priest – and

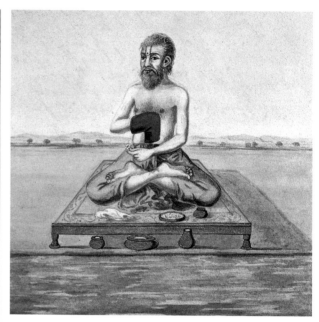

Kapila, one of the earliest known yoga sages, lived in India before 2,500 BCE.

This huge 12th-century statue in Sri Lanka shows the reclining Buddha being translated into nirvana.

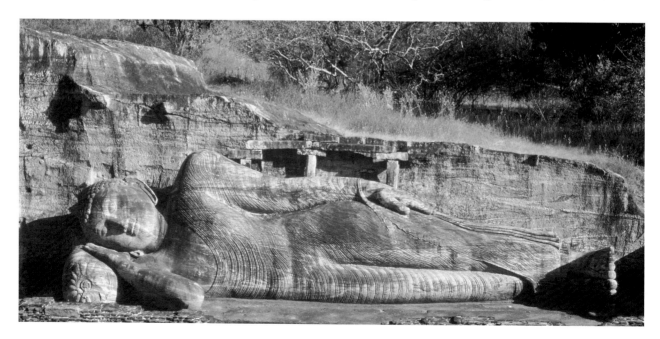

later lived in a forest as an ascetic, where he was taught yoga by a nun, Yogeshwari. He later converted to Islam, then Christianity. He taught that many paths lead to God and came to be regarded as a spiritual genius. He was illiterate, but his talks were collected and published.

Ramakrishna's leading disciple, Swami Vivekenanda, was one of the first Indian yogis to have a major influence in the West. In 1893 he toured the US. As a result of his renown he was fêted as a national hero when he returned to India in 1897 to found the Ramakrishna Mission, now a respected world-wide organization.

The first outstanding yogi to settle in the West was Paramahansa Yogananda, who aimed to reveal "the complete harmony and basic oneness of original yoga and original Christianity as taught by Jesus Christ; and to show that these principles of truth are the common scientific foundation of all true religions." When Yogananda died, in 1952 in Los Angeles, a remarkable statement was issued by the mortuary director of Forest Lawn Memorial Park. In an official letter he declared: "The absence of any visual signs of decay in the dead body of Paramahansa Yogananda offers the most extraordinary case in our experience … no physical disintegration was visible in his body, even 20 days after death." Yogananda's *Autobiography of a Yogi* is now a classic yoga text.

Swami Rama, a yogi from an ashram (place of holy study) in Rishikesh, India, was invited to the US

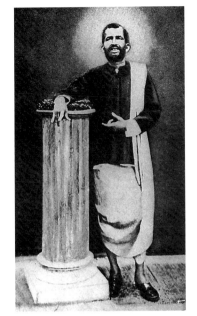

Sri Ramakrishna, a 19th-century yogi and mystic who influenced Swami Vivekenanda.

by the Menninger Institute. Here, doctors Alice and Elmer Green conducted a series of laboratory experiments which demonstrated that he was able to change the temperature of a part of his body at will, and could reduce his heart rate almost to stopping point. Swami Rama founded the Himalayan Institute, also in the US, where research is carried out into the effects of yoga on the body.

Swami Sivananda was a doctor until 1924, when he became a yogi at Rishikesh. He became one of the world's most noted yoga teachers, and many of his followers have played a leading role in promoting yoga worldwide through the Divine Life Society, which he founded in 1936. Among them are Swami Vishnudevananda, based in the US; Swami Sivapremananda, who established centers in Argentina; and Swami Satyananda from Bihar in India.

B.K.S. Iyengar is the most outstanding name in yoga today. He took up yoga in 1934 for health reasons, and by the 1950s he was giving classes and demonstrations in Europe and the US. He has since established active organizations in many countries, and his book, *Light on Yoga*, is published worldwide. His system, Iyengar yoga, takes a more gymnastic approach to the asanas than hatha yoga, for example, and there is less emphasis on breathing and meditation, so it has been criticized as inconsistent with the noncompetitive, holistic basis of traditional yoga.

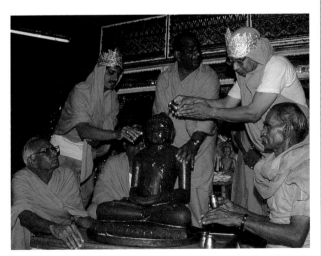

Jain monks bathing a statue of Mahavira, the founder of Jainism. Jainism developed during the 500s BCE and shares many ideas and concepts with yoga. Today, about 2 million people in India practice Jainism.

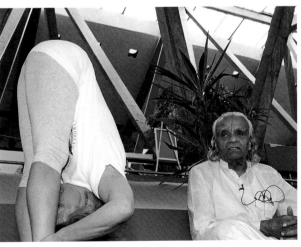

The style of yoga developed by B.K.S. Iyengar, who is seen here at a Yoga Convention in London, England, places a greater emphasis on physical agility than the more traditional schools of yoga.

Objectives

·······················

Many people come to yoga for quite simple reasons. They feel it might help them to cope with stress and be more relaxed, perhaps, or a physician has recommended it as a means of easing their back pain. But lying behind these superficial reasons is almost always a desire for a more fulfilled life. With time, commitment, and effort from the student, yoga can meet all those goals. Anyone who tries the path of yoga will find, if they are serious about it, that their intentions, change along the way. Yoga has its own objectives, which every student must embrace in order to benefit fully.

A leading system of spiritual thought in India, with a great kinship to yoga, is Samkya, which can be translated as "exact knowledge." It is attributed to Kapila, a sage who lived perhaps around 500 BCE. What we should today call Samkya's mission statement declares "Man's supreme goal is the overcoming of suffering." The use of the word "goal" is significant, for it suggests an objective that can be achieved, however difficult.

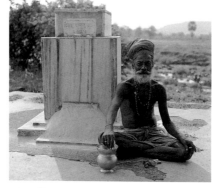

A sadhu or wandering Hindu holy man practicing yoga meditation.

From yoga's earliest days, yogis set themselves to answer the question of how suffering can be overcome. Some 2,000 years ago, the sage Patañjali described yoga as a way of controlling the activities of the mind: "When mind is controlled, Self stays in His native condition. Otherwise He conforms to the nature of mind's activities."

Patañjali's conclusion closely parallels the findings in the mid-20th century of Hans Selye, Professor of External Medicine and Surgery at McGill University, Montreal, Canada, who investigated the effects of prolonged stress on the human mind and body. He found that it results from messages transmitted by the brain that arise from an unusually wide range of sensory inputs. Failure to establish effective control over these multiple messages means that the mind reacts to them willy-nilly, with devastating effects on judgment and action. If people allow themselves to be tossed and turned by uncontrolled signals from the brain, their lives will be in a constant state of uncertainty and stress. Control of the mind is, therefore, considered one of the most effective ways of relieving personal suffering.

A high percentage of illness and disease is known to be connected with or caused by stress. Yoga practices such as stretching and exercising, deep breathing, meditation, and visualization prevent the physical and mental suffering caused by stress, poor posture, lack of exercise, the rigidity that can develop through misuse of the body, aging, and physical disabilities caused by birth defects or accidents.

Patañjali and other sages responded to their perceptions of the causes of suffering by setting themselves the task of finding an approach to life that was calm, controlled, and allowed them to cultivate stillness. They began by considering the wider picture and formulating an ethical or moral approach, recommending followers to be nonviolent, to speak the truth, to refrain from theft, to avoid casual sex, and to be free from greed. The thinking behind these injunctions is that indulging in harmful actions sets up an internal disharmony that causes suffering by damaging people's own lives and the lives of those with whom they come into contact. The sages further enjoined their followers to control their emotions, and not to lose sight of the great teachings of humanity: to be compassionate, to help others, to turn the other cheek.

People studying yoga today find themselves in the happy position of being able to combine the discoveries and teachings of past masters of yoga with many years of detailed scientific research into the needs of mind and body, and their own intuitive approach, to develop an approach or program based on their own requirements and objectives.

YOGA STEP BY STEP

The yoga sages not only made a brilliant analysis of human sorrows but they also devised a whole series of practical steps to overcome them.

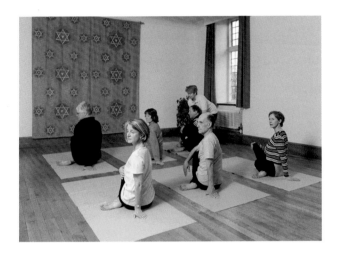

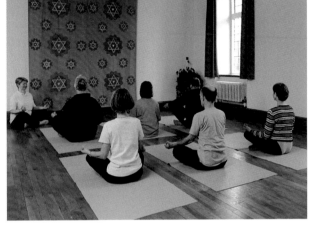

1 *Exercising the body by performing the postures or asanas is the first step undertaken by the newcomer to yoga. Stretching and compressing different parts of the body to make muscles and joints more flexible can overcome many health problems, from RSI (Repetitive Strain Injury) to osteoporosis, and prevent others from developing. In addition, the asanas work on every aspect of personal life, turning strain and irritation into tranquility and contentment, relieving depression and calming hyperactivity.*

2 *Learning how to relax the body and mind rapidly, thoroughly, and at will deepens the beneficial effects of the asanas, and is the second step the beginner learns. Exercise followed by total relaxation removes blockages in the body systems such as the digestive and the nervous systems, and restores the body's normal energy flow.*

3 *Breathing works with exercise and relaxation to stimulate mind and body, promoting self-healing. Breathing practice is an important part of every yoga session since effective breathing strengthens muscles and makes joints stretch further, deepens relaxation, and improves mental control.*

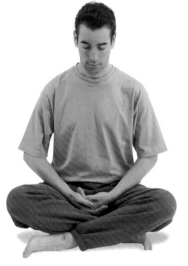

4 *In ancient times yoga was meditation alone. Breathing, relaxation, and asanas were all techniques devised to encourage the dispassionate mental state that is the prelude to meditation. Although these techniques are used much more widely than they once were, meditation and the attainment of states of consciousness in which the mind is elevated above worldly suffering remain the ultimate goals of yoga.*

Classic Schools

....

Yoga is unique among the world's great teachings in that its sages realized long ago that the search for inner peace and understanding may be pursued in manifold ways. As a result, many different schools of yoga have developed at different times during its long history, and new schools continue to arise. People today have a choice between six or more classic school and new styles established by a number of outstanding 20th-century yogis.

One meaning of the word "yoga" is "that which leads the practitioner to the understanding of the oneness, which is the ultimate state of the universe." That understanding may be reached in many different ways – through studying ancient writings, by a life dedicated to helping others with no thought of reward, through deep and prolonged meditation, or, as in hatha yoga, by learning to control the mind through exercising the body, breathing, and practicing concentration. Hatha yoga is most commonly practiced today, but there is a wide choice between the ancient schools, described on these pages, and the newer styles described on pages 16-17.

Hatha yoga: This is the principal form of yoga practiced in the West and its texts emphasize that it is an introductory yoga. It helps beginners to learn, by practicing a number of brilliantly conceptualized techniques, to exert control over body and mind so that they may progress to a deeper stage. The Sanskrit word "hatha" is formed from the sounds "ha" and "tha," which symbolize both the positive and negative electrical forces of the sun and the moon. This is sig-

nificant because a central aspect of the human body is electromagnetism; all body systems have an electrical component, and the heart and brain are regulated by electrical impulses.

Among the techniques of hatha yoga are many of the asanas illustrated in this book. However, the sage Svatmarama, describing some of the major asanas, points out that they are merely a technique for inducing a quiet, contemplative state. The adept yogi should be able to achieve that state of mind without practicing the asanas, and so need use only one posture – the sitting position, for meditation.

Raja yoga: This is often called the king of yogas because "raja," originally a Sanskrit word, means "ruler." One of the leading hatha yoga sages, Svatmarama, declared: "I teach Hatha, only for the sake of Raja Yoga." The Buddha, as depicted in his meditative states, was practicing raja yoga.

This classic school is the yoga of controlling the mind, the yoga, in other words, of scientific meditation, following the steps laid down by Patañjali. They lead the student through a series of stages: first to

THE CLASSIC SCHOOLS OF YOGA
....

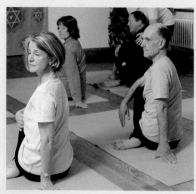

Hatha yoga bridges the gap between the sages and modern practice.

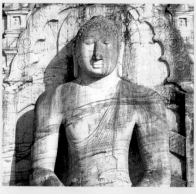

Raja yoga is the yoga of meditation, merging of the Self with the universe.

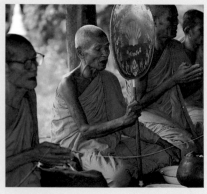

Karma yoga is the yoga of right and selfless action.

effective concentration or single-pointedness, and through a deeper state of contemplation to the ultimate stage, called samadhi. This is a liberating experience in which the consciousness can be said to have risen above the sorrows of human life.

Karma yoga: The Sanskrit word "karma" means both work and destiny. Karma yoga is based on the concept that by being quiet and opening up to our intuition, the actions we have to undertake in life will become clear. These should then be carried out without thought of reward. This does not mean doing good for sanctimonious reasons, but because the right actions, however uncomfortable, may be necessary to advance a situation. Karma yoga is characterized by lack of organization. It is the yoga that exhorts its followers to live for the moment, to "be here now," engendering the state of mind that allows things to happen as they will.

Bhakti yoga: This is also known as the yoga of devotion and will appeal to people who are naturally spiritual or who observe a religion. Yoga is not theistic, for the ultimate force of the universe, known as Brahman, is not thought of as human but as the universal consciousness, the first principle of everything. This, however, does not necessarily mean that worship need play no part in the development of life. Bhakti is the concept of adoration, which plays a major role in many religions. It is very much a personal yoga through which one can achieve higher states of consciousness. The concept of God is used by many people as a focus for meditation.

Jnana yoga: The word "jnana" (pronounced "gyana") means wisdom, and jnana yoga is likely to appeal to people who naturally take an analytical approach to life. Jnana yoga is not exclusively the yoga of the intellect, however, although intellect has its role. Instead, it takes an intuitive route to seeking

FINDING A CLASS

Hatha yoga teachers and classes are easy to find in many countries of the world, and it is possible to find groups practicing mantra yoga and bhakti yoga in the West as well as the East. To practice the other forms of yoga described here will be more difficult, although major yoga institutions and societies should have information.

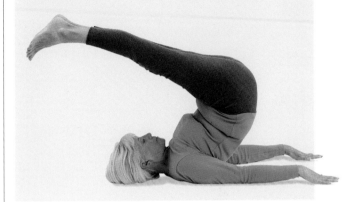

answers to the great questions of life, such as how to discriminate between the real and the un-real. Jnana yoga is often practiced in groups, who read and discuss the classic texts of yoga.

Mantra yoga: This is the yoga associated with chanting monks in Tibetan monasteries. It involves raising the consciousness by chanting, aloud or to oneself, sounds, words, or sentences called mantras. The repetition of a mantra is central to Tibetan and some other schools of meditation. Chanting is a natural and enjoyable human activity, a way of expressing emotion. The idea behind chanting a mantra is that it assists concentration which may elevate the mind.

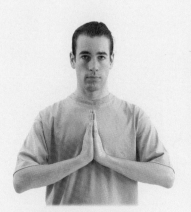

Bhakti yoga is the yoga of devotion to a deity.

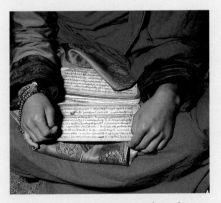

Jnana yoga is the yoga of wisdom and knowledge.

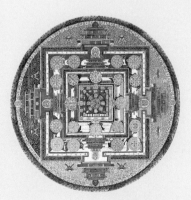

Mantra yoga involves the use of divine symbols and sacred sounds.

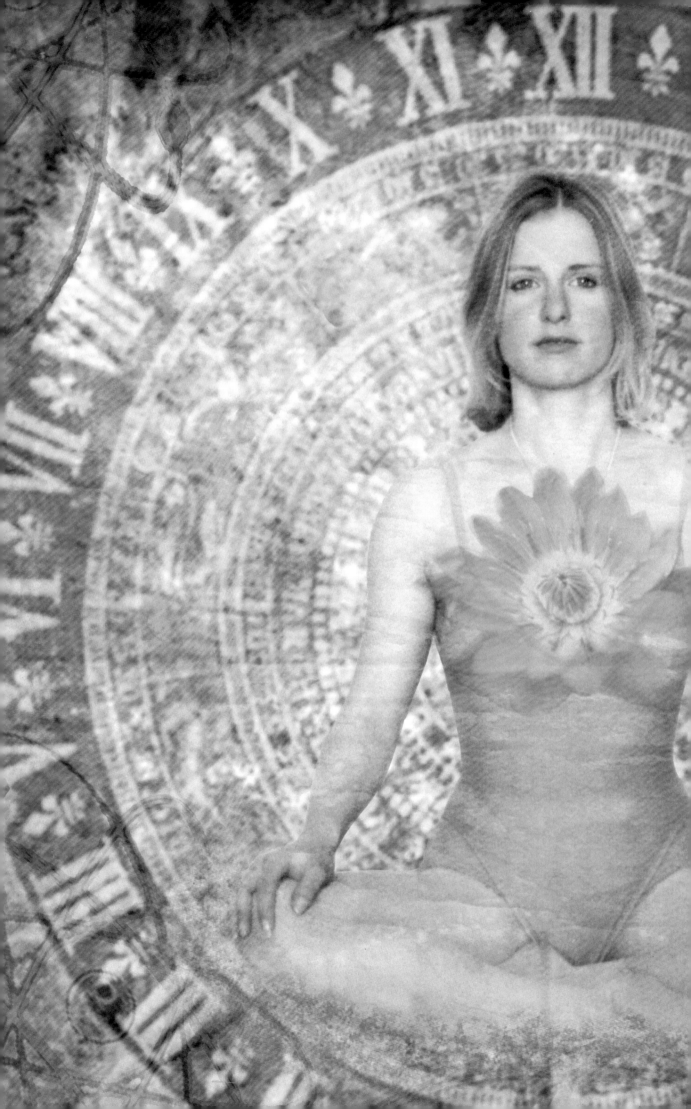

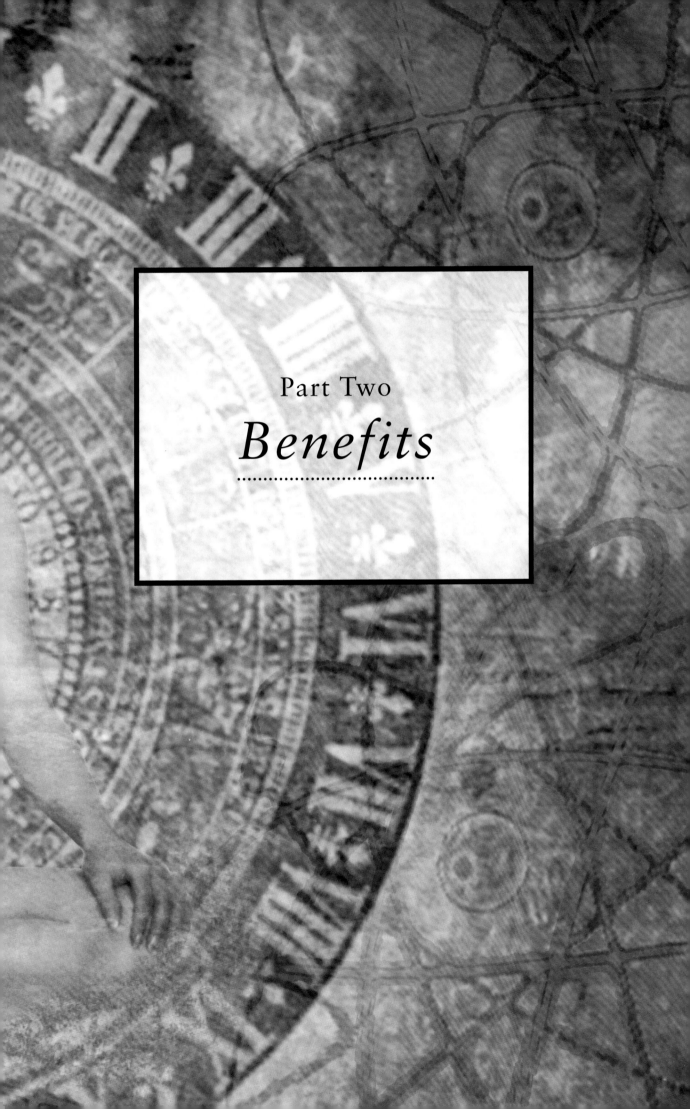

Part Two
Benefits

Benefits of Yoga

....

The body is an energy system with close interplay between breathing, heart beat, and brain function. Yoga provides a maintenance service for that system. Rightly described as "the heart of healing," yoga also provides a harmonizing process that leaves no part of the body untouched.

Working from the premise that "Life is breath, breath is life," yoga places great emphasis on making the breathing deep, rhythmic, and effective. Respiration, the thinking goes, is not just a matter of exchanging gases, it is also the body's pumping system. The diaphragm (the large muscle that stretches across the body between the chest and the abdomen) forms a cone during inhalation, which acts as the piston of body energy. To function effectively it depends upon the movement of the lower ribs, and these depend upon posture and natural breathing to work properly themselves.

Respiration is the source of oxygen and other gases that fuel the body. They penetrate the lung tissues to dissolve in the blood, and they are pumped along with other nutrients through tiny capillaries to nourish the extremities of the body, and through major arteries to the great organs, such as the brain. To work effectively the brain requires not only effective oxygenation but also a rhythmic flow of electromagnetic energy, generated by the heart and transported by the nerves. Without these, essential thoughts and messages will be muddled and negative, and the body will suffer from tiredness and incapacity.

Yoga asanas and yogic breathing stimulate the nervous system, clearing the body's electromagnetic energy pathways to and from the brain. This is one channel through which breathing affects outlook. Poor breathing may not always be the cause of low spirits, but shallow or irregular breathing invariably accompany attacks of depression and other mood swings and disorders. The heart, like the breath, responds to the mind's perceptions of life.

Electrocardiograms show the damage caused by habitually negative thoughts, and conversely the healing process that may be brought about by more positive ones.

Even the bony skeleton of the body is affected by the mental and physical harmony that yoga can bring about. Bone, like other tissue, is constantly renewing itself, and the body's electromagnetic energy plays a central part in this renewal, so yoga helps maintain bone density. The joints require balanced use if they are to work well. The interplay between mental calmness, free flow of the breath, and harmonized movement, provided by yoga, helps to maintain this balance.

Because of its emphasis on balanced stretching and exercise, yoga can be used to prevent and ease many painful conditions caused by the overuse of joints and limbs, from hamstring and other sports injuries to a frozen shoulder. It can also provide short-term remedies for complaints caused by stress, including tension headaches and hyperventilation (fast, shallow breathing).

Yoga encourages heart and brain to function freely, unhampered by stress. Although it can take long and regular practice to restore some of the damage caused by years of neglect, beginners can take heart from the knowledge that improvement can be seen in many aspects of body function and mental outlook after just a few sessions. In the long term, however, yoga brings about emotional control, resulting in a peaceful state of mind and a calm lifestyle, and more effective functioning of every part of the body.

The tree posture is one of many asanas that improve balance and coordination.

BODY MAINTENANCE THROUGH YOGA

Improved appearance, through better posture and muscle and skin tone, follows the dedicated practice of yoga. The bones are strengthened and the joints become more mobile. It can seem astonishing how much more flexible the body is and how much more positive one's outlook becomes with a few months of regular yoga practice. To achieve these benefits, however, as much attention must be given to breathing and relaxation as to the asanas.

Fewer and less intense headaches result from stretching and exercising the spine, relieving pressure on the cervical vertebrae (bones of the neck), from improved blood circulation and reduced blood pressure, and from regular relaxation brought about by exercise combined with breathing and meditation.

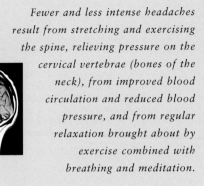

Improved oxygen supply to the blood and the rhythmic flow of electromagnetic energy along the nerves result in better concentration and clarity of thought.

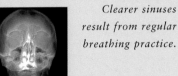

Clearer sinuses result from regular breathing practice.

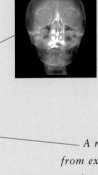

The tendency to back pain is reduced since the spine becomes more flexible due to frequent stretching and mobility exercises.

A relaxed posture results from exercising regularly and improvements in balance.

Digestion is improved since effective breathing stimulates the whole digestive system and abdominal massage stimulates the organs inside the abdomen. Stretching and exercising the abdominal muscles keeps the stomach flat.

Breathing deepens and becomes rhythmic, relieving disorders such as hyperventilation and asthma, or making them less likely to develop. The heart benefits from regular exercise and effective breathing, which stimulate blood circulation and reduces blood pressure.

The hip joints are kept flexible and mobile by regular exercise and correct carriage of the upper body. Improved electromagnetic energy flow prevents bone loss, making hip replacement and thinning bones less likely in later life.

The knee and ankle joints remain supple because of better posture in the upper body and regular exercise.

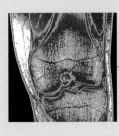

Balance is improved by better posture and regular exercise.

Internal Peace

·····························

Most people in industrialized countries experience a glimpse of yogic peace at the beginning of a vacation. Feeling under strain from the pressures of life, the break from everyday routines to a place where there is sunshine and a peaceful beach has been anticipated with much pleasure. After the additional stress of the journey, most vacationers are soon lying doing nothing. For a short while, mind and body exalt in the wonderful sensation of just being.

Curiously, this euphoric state is the result of a form of concentration. The mind builds up an overwhelming desire to experience a state of peace and a situation has been created in which that can happen, so it does. Other forms of concentration come about in moments of crisis. One example was reported in the British newspapers a number of years ago. A mother discovered to her horror that her small child had been trapped under the back wheels of an automobile, so she rushed over and lifted up the back of the vehicle in order to release the child. At any other time she would not have believed herself capable of such a feat of strength, but the urgency of the moment pushed away any negative thoughts in her mind.

It is hardly practical, however, for most people to keep going off on vacation, and for those who could, the effect would gradually diminish. And since vacations and emergencies come along only infrequently to bring about total concentration, the mind needs training to bring the chattering thoughts under control. Yoga provides that necessary training.

A large part of yoga consists of practicing the asanas – the Sanskrit word used in yoga for a position or posture involving the body. The original asanas were a number of sitting positions in which yogis meditated. As yoga developed, many thousands more were created. The asanas are executed in a comfortably upright position, reflecting the body's posture. When they are carried out correctly they ensure that the lungs work efficiently, so that the breathing is free

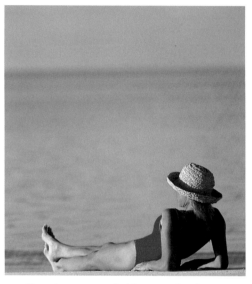

Yoga is a more reliable way of inducing inner peace than a vacation.

and operates rhythmically, helping to stimulate the heart, and that the digestive system and the associated glands and organs operate efficiently. Training the posture affects brain functioning, strengthening the power of clear thinking and increasing concentration.

In recent years research has established that the human body functions effectively on numerous interweaving rhythms, of which breathing is just one. Research into sleep patterns has established that dreams occur approximately every 90 minutes, though people are unaware of most of their dreams. Now it has been shown that people tend to daydream on the same rhythmical pattern. The stomach exhibits a pattern of contractions related to the need for food. In one experiment a group of people instructed to eat snacks whenever they wished ate according to the same pattern – every 90 minutes.

For many centuries yogis have known that each nostril tends to be used alternately, that is, one nostril engorges slightly, while the other allows free passage of air – and this pattern reverses roughly every 90 minutes. Now, researchers have concluded that this breathing pattern is related to the dominance of the brain hemispheres: research in the US has indicated that people relax more easily when breathing mainly through the left nostril, which has a relationship with the right hemisphere of the brain. There are links between these cycles and the 24-hour circadian rhythm – the basic human biorhythm. In the practice of yoga, working within these natural rhythms is the key to establishing a state of inner peace.

THE BODY CLOCK

Humans are seasonal creatures and many of the body's systems vary in a rhythmic way, in cycles that fluctuate from a year to the numerous twice-daily or circadian rhythms that govern most of the body's systems. The whole body, even down to individual cells, is governed by rhythms; the liver cells show a circadian rhythm in the rate at which they break down drugs, and the cells of the kidneys in the rate at which they excrete them. Cyclical variations have also been measured in the blood pressure and the diameter of the air passages in the lungs. There is much to learn about human biorhythms, but researchers believe that information about light, darkness, temperature, and other factors is transmitted along the nerves from the sense organs to the brain, where it may act to synchronize one of the body's master clocks, the pituitary gland, which controls the output of hormones from a number of glands.

Pineal gland: *The cycle of sleep and wakefulness is influenced by the level of melatonin, secreted by the pineal gland in the brain, which is stimulated by darkness and suppressed by light.*

Pituitary gland: *The body's internal clock is regulated by hormones released into the bloodstream by the endocrine glands. The output of these glands is controlled by the pituitary gland in the brain.*

Kidneys: *The cycle of sleep and wakefulness is influenced by the hormone cortisol secreted by the adrenal glands, which is low at bedtime and high early in the morning.*

Ovaries: *A hormone released roughly every 28 days stimulates the ovaries to produce egg follicles and release an egg.*

MAINTAINING HARMONY

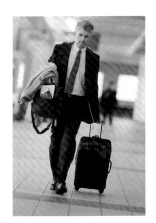

International travel disrupts our body clock.

The demands of modern life do not always coincide with the rhythms of the body. Working late, doing all-night shifts, and fast travel across the datelines all disturb the body's biological clock. This can cause symptoms of ill health that vary with the individual but may include tiredness, headaches, tension, irritability, and a degree of mental confusion.

Total relaxation is the best way to deal with these symptoms. On returning home immediately after a late shift or a long international flight, change into comfortable, loose-fitting clothes, lay a towel or a mat on the floor and relax totally as described on pages 72–73 for at least 10 minutes. Concentrate on easing the tensions in mind and body, and on breathing quietly and rhythmically.

It can take some days for the body to readjust to jet lag. The symptoms will ease if you remember to stop regularly, sit somewhere quiet and breathe slowly for two or three minutes, emphasizing the out-breaths. This stimulates the blood circulation and relieves mental and physical tension. Also continue to relax totally once or twice a day for at least 10 minutes. The combination of both types of relaxation is a gentle way of exercising control over mind and body to banish physical discomfort and mental confusion, and help restore harmony.

Periodic relaxation sessions relieve symptoms caused by biorhythm disturbance.

Healing Process

·······································

When you buy a new machine, a manual comes with it giving instructions on how to use it and what to do if anything goes wrong with it. Unfortunately, however, people are born with no useful manual attached to their bodies. Since the dawn of consciousness, therefore, generations of physicians have had to try to deduce from observation and experiment how to look after the body, how it works, and how to repair it when it malfunctions.

Much is known about how the human body and brain work, but there is much still to discover. Few people pause to consider that the body and the mind are still undergoing a process of development that has been taking place for millions of years.

Yoga teachers repeatedly urge their students to become aware of their own bodies and so attempt to train them to become in tune with this evolutionary process. The advantages of greater awareness are diverse. Not only do students become more flexible and proficient at performing the yoga postures but they also feel more fulfilled, with a deepened capacity to cope with the problems that everyday life throws up. Practicing yoga helps the mind perceive these problems in perspective, as challenges. This helps the students to see that the development of each individual's life is bound up with the way in which they are confronted and resolved.

Yoga teaches that life is the action and reaction of pulsations, the intricate interplay of a vast number of energy fields. These energy fields should function in complex harmony, and illness is the result of a breakdown of this harmony. On analyzing this breakdown, modern medicine will often conclude that some body ingredient is missing, or in short supply, or overabundant. Drugs will often be the remedy chosen in an interventionist attempt to correct the balance. Yoga works in a more holistic way, attempting to understand why the imbalance has occurred, then using the body's internal systems to restore the balance.

In his compendium of hatha yoga, the *Hathapradipika*, Svatmarama, a sage who lived in the 13th or 14th century, writes about illnesses such as heart problems and asthma, which he diagnoses as arising from the incorrect practice of yoga. Svatmarama was writing for a limited readership of yogis and might be expected to give detailed instructions for combating illnesses by performing different asanas or special techniques. Instead, he writes, "Whenever any region is affected by disease one should contemplate upon the 'Vayu' situated in that region." Vayu can be translated as "energy fields." He adds, "With concentrated mind one should meditate upon it [that is, the disease] and should fill the lungs by inhaling. Then a complete exhalation should be effortfully performed according to one's capacity."

There is evidence that sprains and fractures can benefit from the release of energy that yoga encourages. The example of Yehudi Menuhin mentioned on page 10 is only one example. A fracture causes an imbalance of energy in the affected area such that the electrical receptivity of the injury site is reduced. It has been suggested that yogic breathing and visualization exercises may help to restore the flow of neuroelectric energy to the injured area.

Yoga unites the benefits of performing the asanas with breathing and with meditation and visualization (concentrating the energy of the mind on a visual image with positive associations) to create a uniquely powerful healing force.

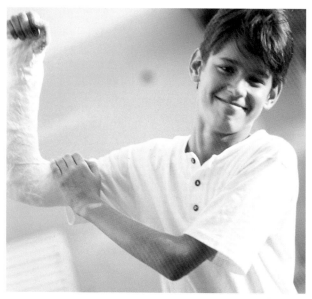

Yoga techniques are employed to alleviate many illnesses and even to treat injuries.

HEALING THROUGH YOGA

Yogis believe that *citta* (mental activities) and *prana* (the life force) run together, that the perceptible form which the functioning of prana takes is respiration, and that diseases result from an obstruction in its natural functioning. Yogis believe that by practicing slow respiration, stopping the breath for shorter or longer periods and directing the mind to the part of the body where pain is felt, the disease-producing obstruction is removed and the natural functioning of prana is restored in that part of the body.

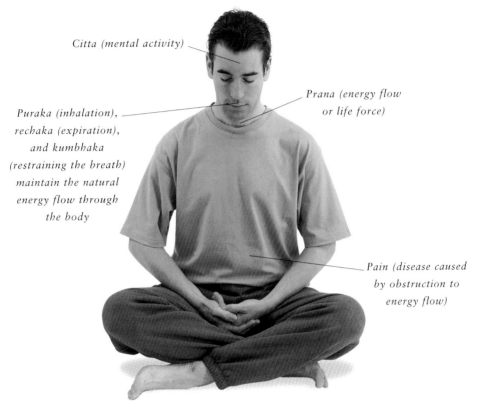

Citta (mental activity)

Prana (energy flow or life force)

Puraka (inhalation), rechaka (expiration), and kumbhaka (restraining the breath) maintain the natural energy flow through the body

Pain (disease caused by obstruction to energy flow)

COMPLETE RELAXATION (SHAVASANA)

The art of relaxation is an important part of hatha yoga, for complete relaxation eliminates the stresses and tensions which block the flow of prana, or energy, around the body, resulting in pain and illness. Calming the mind through relaxation is a form of preventive medicine since it results in a more balanced outlook and so prevents stresses from arising.

MEDITATION

Hatha yoga encourages its followers to practice meditation – withdrawing mind from body (though maintaining an awareness of it), and concentrating on something nonphysical, such as the concept of peace – as a way of easing tensions in the mind and the body, so preventing and curing disease. An Australian psychiatrist, the late Dr. Ainslie Meares, used meditation techniques to treat cancers.

VISUALIZATION

Yoga teachers emphasize the importance of visualization – concentrating on an image of, for instance, a tranquil rural landscape – to stimulate the body's internal systems. Visualization is believed to ease bodily and mental tensions and so stimulate health. An American cancer specialist, Dr. Carl Simonton, has become famous for his use of visualization to overcome disease.

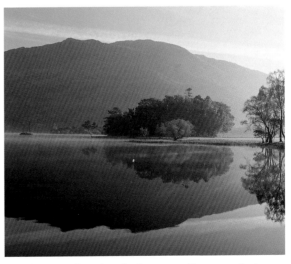

Planning short breaks for tranquil contemplation during the year benefits mental and physical health.

Mental and Physical Approach

The development of the human species seems little short of a miracle. Modern anthropologists have been able to trace its physical development from Homo erectus, *the earliest humanoids, using carbon-dating and other techniques. The bodies of* Homo erectus *developed in association with a deepening of consciousness and the emergence of self-awareness. Hunter-gatherers needed to communicate and so, probably slowly and awkwardly, physical and mental changes produced language.*

Reconstructions of *Homo erectus* look so different from modern people that it has been hard for some to accept that these alien creatures are their direct ancestors, and even more difficult to believe that *Homo sapiens* evolved from single-celled creatures that emerged eons ago from Earth's primordial soup. Considering the diversity of predators that inhabited Earth throughout the evolution of modern humans, it seems impossible that this fragile species should have survived, let alone multiplied to dominate all others. Physical strength and capability cannot provide the only explanation,

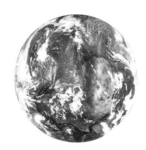

The evolution of consciousness ensured the survival of the human species on Earth.

for early humans could scarcely defend themselves against the whole variety of tusked, clawed, armor-plated, and flying creatures that sought to prey on them. The conclusion must be that their survival owes much to the slow but sure development of what is called consciousness, or, in yoga, atman.

It was the power of intuitive thought that brought yoga to the respected position it occupies today among the many branches of Hindu philosophy. It was, for example, the meditational practices of jnana yoga, the yoga of wisdom, that produced the Upanishads, the 2,500-year-old yoga

BRAIN DEVELOPMENT

The earliest humanoids were shorter than modern humans. As they evolved they grew taller and walked upright, and their brain increased remarkably in size.

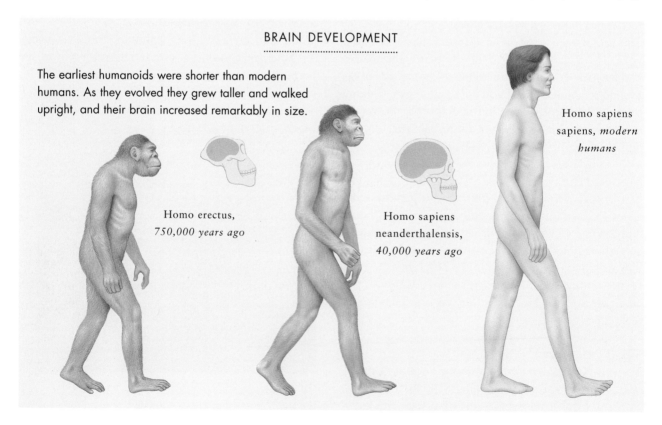

Homo erectus, *750,000 years ago*

Homo sapiens neanderthalensis, *40,000 years ago*

Homo sapiens sapiens, *modern humans*

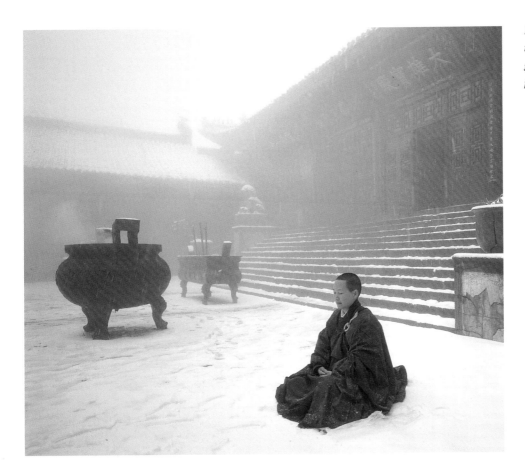

Buddhist monks harness the power of yoga to gain control over physical discomfort.

scriptures. The *Katha Upanishad*, the story of a boy granted three wishes by Yama, god of death, elaborates on the concept of atman. It is found, says the Upanishad, deep in the heart. It is the eternal in every person which cannot die. The atman is everyone's own higher self, and their goal is to seek it through yoga. It can be found when the senses and the mind are still, and reason rests in silence. This calm steadiness of the senses is yoga.

In seeking to describe this mysterious force that lies at the root of everything, the sages of ancient times had to resort to negatives, "The one without a second," "Not this – not this." Ancient Eastern texts suggest that the First Cause, the Prime Mover that created the universe, expresses itself in consciousness. If this is so, the survival and evolution of humankind must have arisen from an interplay between consciousness and the developing body. As the mind grew, so the body refined itself, changing its form to fit it for the new, developing role of human beings on Earth.

It is often asserted that concepts such as the atman are all in the mind. However, nothing is wholly mental just as nothing can be wholly physical. From the earliest stages of yoga thought, recognition was given to the special role of breathing – the part played by the breath of life in energizing body and mind. And every aspect of yoga is an interplay between mind and body, whose aim is to liberate the flow of energy upon which all thought and all life depends.

THE AGE-OLD QUESTION

An Eastern text, more than 2,000 years old, expresses an age-old puzzle:

From where do we come? By what do we live?
Where shall we find peace at last?
What power governs the duality
Of pleasure and pain by which we are driven?

Time, nature, necessity, accident,
Elements, energy, intelligence –
None of these can be the First Cause.
They are effects, whose only purpose is
To help the Self rise above pleasure and pain.

Shvetashvatara Upanishad

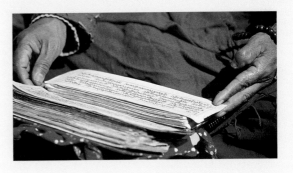

Commitment

....

Deciding to take up yoga means making a commitment to improve the quality of one's mental and physical life. The classic yoga texts stress the importance of practicing in a tranquil place at regular times. Today, the psychological significance of this approach is clear, for it is now understood that to repeat an activity at set intervals accustoms the mind to accept it as part of everyday life. Like the sages of ancient times, yoga teachers today recommend setting aside regular hours to practice hatha yoga and to meditate in a suitably quiet place.

Developing the self-discipline to practice regularly is part of yoga, for discipline is, essentially, practicing something until it becomes habitual. At first this may seem off-putting, adding another burden to what is, for many people, already an over-demanding lifestyle. However, when what is being practiced produces benefits, the discipline quickly stops being a chore and becomes a natural and worthwhile habit.

Ideally yoga sessions need to take place every day at about the same time. Many asanas exercise the digestive organs, and for this the stomach and intestines need to be as empty as possible, so it is best not to have eaten for at least two hours before practice. A session might

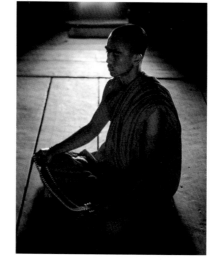

A period of withdrawal from life's demands is an ancient means of restoring one's self.

last from about half an hour initially up to perhaps two hours once the beginner's stage is passed. Yoga practice is energizing, not tiring, so people who like to be up early in the morning prefer to practice before breakfast. Others find it an excellent relaxant and pick-me-up in the early evening. People who work from home often find late morning the best time.

Although it seems a simple enough project to set aside an hour or so at the same time every day to practice yoga, modern lifestyles make it almost impossible for some people to do so. People whose work involves frequent and often unpredictable travel or overtime sessions, and anyone with a young family, finds it scarcely possible to organize a single meal for themselves at the same time each day.

The best way to approach this problem is to begin by scaling it down, planning one or two practice sessions at the same time each week. Most people can find an hour on a Saturday or Sunday morning, or late in the evening once or twice a week. Late evening, when most people are tired, is not an ideal time for practice, but for some people it is a good way of unwinding at the end of a very long and stressful day, and they sleep more deeply as a result. Stick to the scaled-down plan zealously and the benefits will be so obvious that making more time for practice moves close to the top of the list of priorities. A daily sequence of asanas, lasting at least 15 minutes and preferably nearer half an hour, will make an immense difference to life.

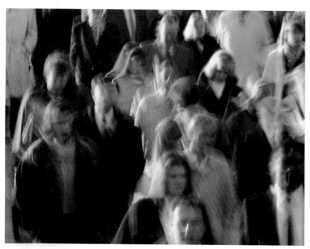

A morning yoga session makes the day's events easier to deal with.

For beginners, the most important objective is to practice regularly. Brush aside worries about tasks unfinished or not yet begun – yoga works to clear the mind of daily preoccupations and students often find they can organize their lives more efficiently as a result. Resist the temptation to miss practice because "something comes up" by rescheduling the unforeseen event. If something unavoidable does intervene, fit in the practice after it.

Finding somewhere quiet can be difficult. The world is full of underused quiet places, however, such as bedrooms, bathrooms, balconies, and gardens, family rooms when children are sleeping, unused offices and meeting rooms, even a washroom. It is possible to learn to ignore incidental noise, such as aircraft and traffic, so for many a quiet place is simply somewhere where other people cannot immediately get hold of them.

EQUIPMENT FOR YOGA

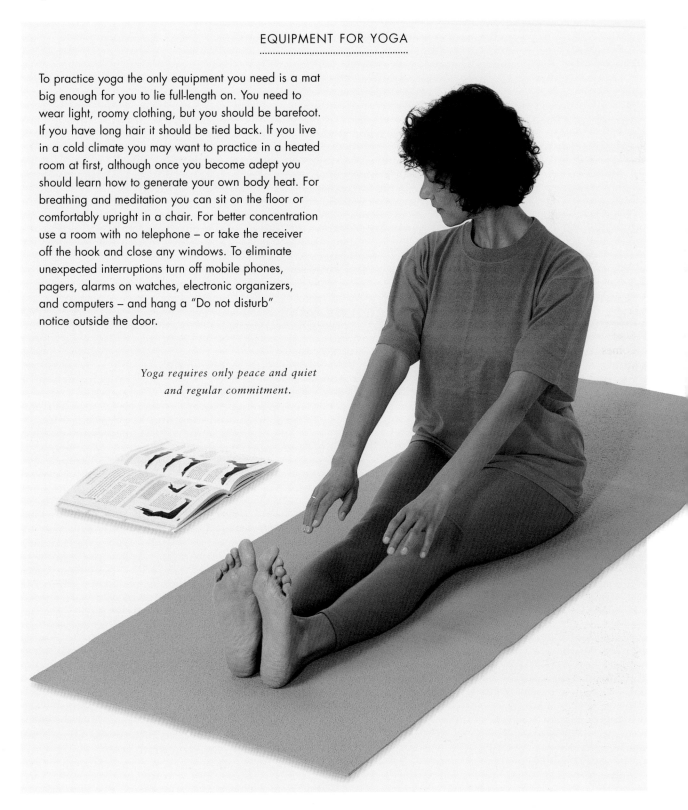

To practice yoga the only equipment you need is a mat big enough for you to lie full-length on. You need to wear light, roomy clothing, but you should be barefoot. If you have long hair it should be tied back. If you live in a cold climate you may want to practice in a heated room at first, although once you become adept you should learn how to generate your own body heat. For breathing and meditation you can sit on the floor or comfortably upright in a chair. For better concentration use a room with no telephone – or take the receiver off the hook and close any windows. To eliminate unexpected interruptions turn off mobile phones, pagers, alarms on watches, electronic organizers, and computers – and hang a "Do not disturb" notice outside the door.

Yoga requires only peace and quiet and regular commitment.

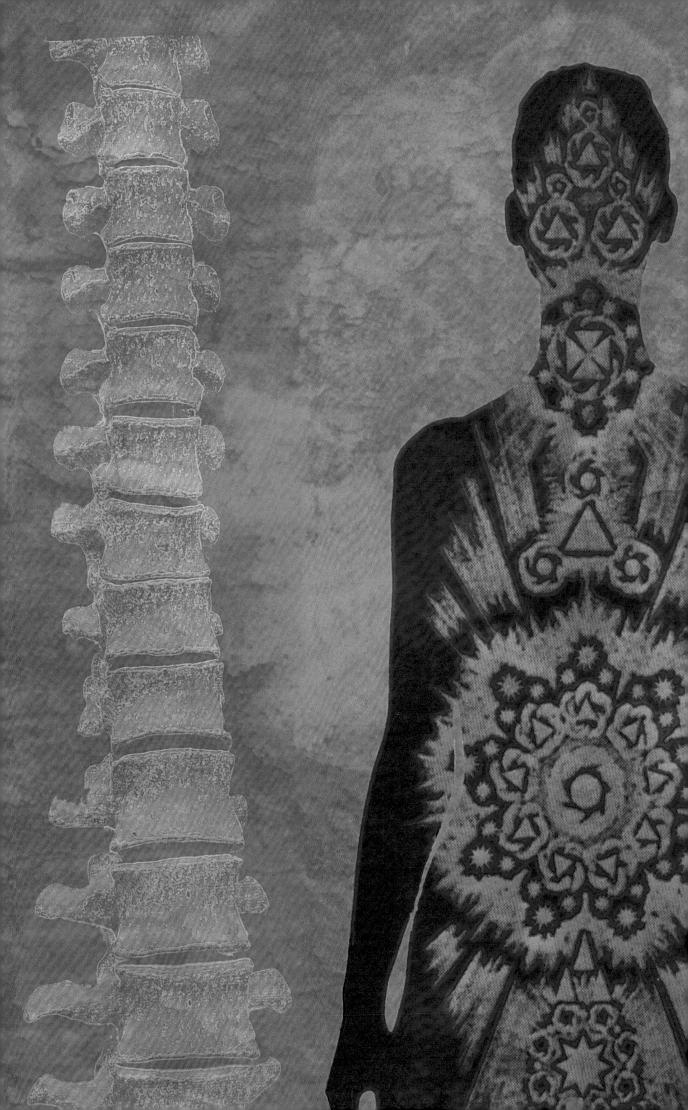

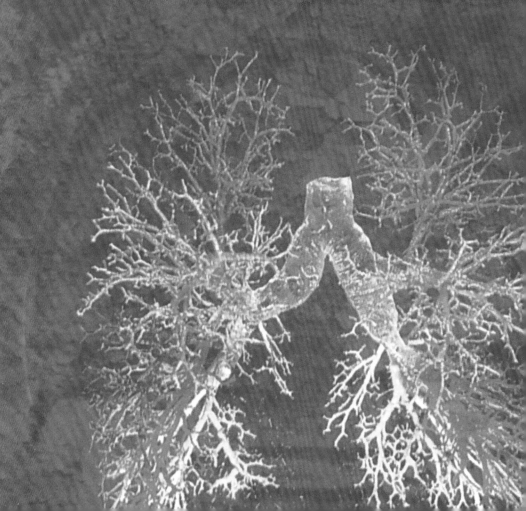

Part Three

Anatomy
and Posture

Yoga and the Body

....

Some early yoga texts liken the body to a chariot, pulled by horses (the senses), and guided by the Self as charioteer who, aided by the mind, sees that all three operate in harmony. What fuels the body is energy, and what is astonishing is that its energy is directed to maintaining itself. Every human cell feeds itself, grows, excretes waste products, moves, and reproduces. These activities make each cell and the whole organism dependent on its environment, for cells take their energy from and return it to their surroundings.

What distinguishes living things from inanimate objects is that all life acts as though it desires to perpetuate its existence. "A cell sets out to maintain itself as though acting in accordance with some design to which it subscribes... it is purposive and resourceful," wrote a Harley Street physician, Dr. Kenneth Walker, in 1942. The immune response, through which the body produces agents we call antibodies to destroy disease-causing organisms that penetrate the body's defences, is an excellent example to support this idea of purpose and direction.

The overwhelming dominance of modern scientific ideas and medical advances makes us forget that human existence is totally integrated with the life force, or prana. This is the catalyst that drives the body to function as a purposive, cooperative whole, one that is so sophisticated that we have not yet begun to understand it. Yoga works holistically with body and mind to reinforce the prana. Through breathing, stretching and exercise, relaxation, and meditation yoga stimulates the immune system and the other maintenance systems, and tries to create a state of harmony between body, mind, and the external world.

Well-maintained and balanced according to the perceptions of yoga, the body can function effectively without much outside intervention, preventing illness from occurring and healing itself when injured. This is not to deny the physician, the surgeon, or the medical researcher their role when body systems malfunction and breakdowns occur, but healers play a subordinate role to that of our own long-term responsibility for our body.

Part of that responsibility is to supply the body with everything it needs from the environment for optimum functioning. These are simple: enough unpolluted air, supplied through practicing effective breathing, and a nutritious diet.

No two bodies are alike, however. Some people are double-jointed and many have one leg that is very slightly longer than the other. Such differences mean that no single program or way of practicing the asanas can be suitable for everyone. Yoga is a slow process of self-realization and all students need to assess their capabilities and to experiment with many yoga styles, techniques, and postures until they find a path that is right for them.

The yoga belief is that the body is to be cooperated with; that if encouraged, it will serve us well; that if we trust it, it will not let us down. Those who deride yoga's approach to the body should ask themselves whether we have discovered all there is to know about the forces behind the universe. The answer we give is that we have hardly begun the great voyage of discovery.

No school of yoga is right for everyone. Each body is different and every person must search for the right path.

MAINTAINING THE BODY'S MAJOR ORGANS

Like the rest of the body, the important organs within the abdomen need to exercise, but they cannot move in the way that the limbs or the neck can. They are stimulated by the movements of the body in exercise – particularly by the up-and-down movements of the diaphragm during breathing. Yoga teachers call this passive exercise of the abdominal organs "massage." The organs within the rib cage – the lungs and the heart – can similarly be exercised by massage.

Massaging the abdominal organs through breathing and other movements benefits them mainly by speeding the supply of blood to and from them, so that waste products are quickly removed and essential nutrients are in constant supply. It also stimulates the involuntary, wavelike motions of the digestive organs – the stomach, intestines, bladder, and rectum – and the action of glands such as the pancreas, which supply enzymes used to digest food.

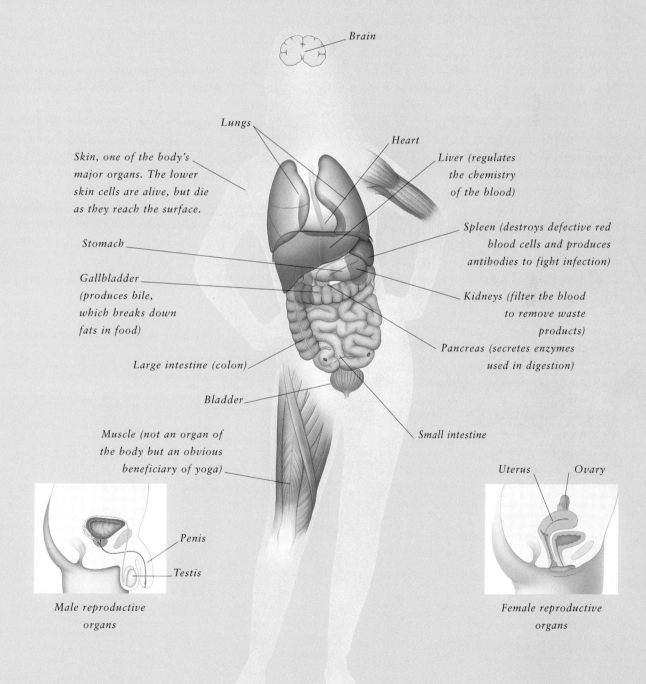

Brain

Lungs

Heart

Liver (regulates the chemistry of the blood)

Skin, one of the body's major organs. The lower skin cells are alive, but die as they reach the surface.

Spleen (destroys defective red blood cells and produces antibodies to fight infection)

Stomach

Gallbladder (produces bile, which breaks down fats in food)

Kidneys (filter the blood to remove waste products)

Large intestine (colon)

Pancreas (secretes enzymes used in digestion)

Bladder

Muscle (not an organ of the body but an obvious beneficiary of yoga)

Small intestine

Uterus   Ovary

Penis

Testis

Male reproductive organs

Female reproductive organs

Chakras

. . . .

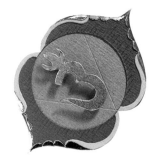

The yoga concept of the life force, expressed by the Sanskrit word "prana," is beyond our understanding. It includes the gases of the atmosphere and the force of electromagnetism. It is the life force that powers the human mind and body. Yet it is much greater than any and all of these. It is the force of consciousness itself.

The miracle of human energy resides in the concept of the chakras. A chakra is a wheel or vortex of energy and it is postulated that the chakras occupy a meridian running from the groin to the top of the head, along the line of the spinal column. The chakras align not only with the spine but also with the sites of important endocrine glands. The glands in this group all release hormones directly into the bloodstream that affect the entire body, from its major organs to its individual cells. And the chakras align with the major plexes of the part of the nervous system that controls unconscious functions, such as the heart beat, and the secretions of the endocrine glands.

In natural health these energy centers respond to the body's energy needs from moment to moment. However, factors ranging from poor posture to inferior breathing and unhealthy food can damage their ability to function. This brings about a range of problems, from lethargy to symptoms of ill health. The yoga approach to breathing is designed to stimulate the natural functioning of the chakras. By working on the body to improve posture and encouraging healthy eating, yoga promotes an effective flow of energy through all parts of the body.

Human energy is still a mystery and the presence of the chakras is not yet proven scientifically, but there is increasing medical and scientific interest in the concept. The simple tests illustrated opposite also indicate their presence. One test is carried out on the site of the manipura chakra, the second on the site of the anahata chakra. These two chakras lie either side of the diaphragm, the body's energy pump, and this accounts for the remarkable changes in energy levels before and after deep breathing revealed by the test.

THE TRADITIONAL CHAKRA SYSTEM

. . . .

The sages perceived the universe as vibrating with the energy of life or prana, and its vibrations may be understood aurally as a seven-note interval of music, or visually as the spectrum of seven colors. The traditional chakra system illustrated in the ancient yoga texts and reproduced here was designed to help yogis memorize the form of the universe. The chakras are the six centers spaced along the nadi (channel), called the sushumna, and the seventh at the top. Each chakra represents a node (the point on a plant stem from which branches or leaves grow). Two curved paths called the ida and the pingala emerge from the lowest center and terminate in the sixth.

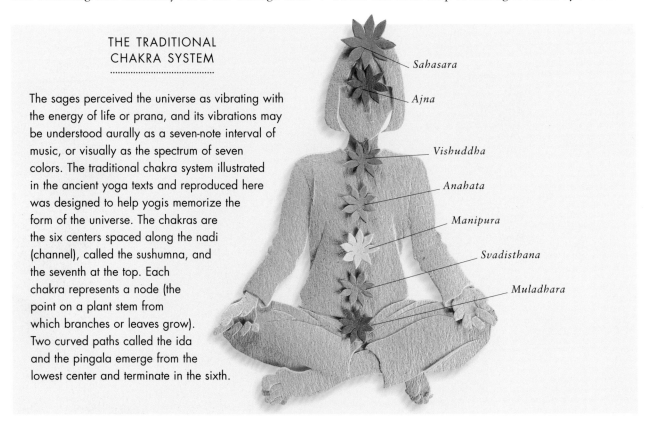

Sahasara

Ajna

Vishuddha

Anahata

Manipura

Svadisthana

Muladhara

TESTING FOR THE CHAKRAS

If you have not been active before you test the manipura chakra (steps 1-2), you will need to generate energy to increase the muscle tone. The pressure of your fingers will be stronger than the force in the area you press and the muscle tone will be weak. Deep breathing stimulates the energy in this area, so when you press it the second time, the pressure of your fingers will be less than the energy field.

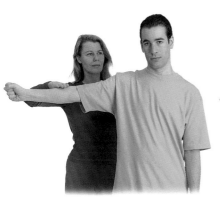 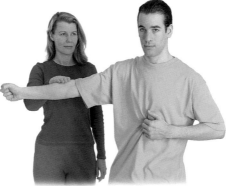 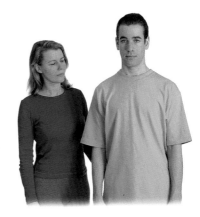

1 *Stand with the feet a little apart and extend your right arm out to the side with the fist clenched to tense the muscles. The second person stands behind you and presses on one of the muscles of your extended arm to check the tone.*

2 *Keeping your right arm extended and the fist clenched, make talons with the fingers of your left hand and press into your abdomen, just above your navel. The second person, still standing behind you, should now press on one of the muscles of your right arm and will feel that it has gone very weak.*

3 *Drop your arms and take half a dozen deep breaths in and out, keeping your chest and abdomen still. Feel your bottom (false or floating) ribs to check that they are rising and falling.*

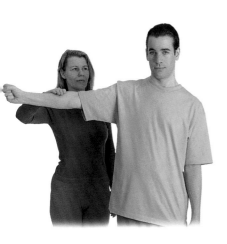 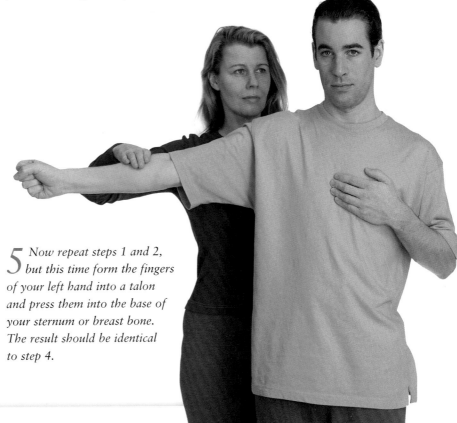

4 *Now extend your right arm again and clench the fist to tense the arm muscles. The second person should check the muscle tone once more and should find that it has greatly increased.*

5 *Now repeat steps 1 and 2, but this time form the fingers of your left hand into a talon and press them into the base of your sternum or breast bone. The result should be identical to step 4.*

Nadis

....

The idea that the human body contains an intricate pattern of channels along which flows life energy has been advanced for thousands of years. The Chinese called these channels meridians and evolved a form of healing, called acupuncture, in which pressure applied at particular points along these meridians could stimulate health. Yogic texts describe a similar energy system in which life energy, or prana, flows along channels called nadis.

Although acupuncture is now practiced in the West by many doctors, no one really knows why it is so often effective. The idea of energy flowing along channels within the body has raised much controversy among Western medical scientists and is often derided. It is interesting, however, that on March 6, 1936 the influential *British Medical Journal* included a report by Sir Thomas Lewis, who claimed to have identified a third nervous system beside the central and autonomic nervous systems. He described it as too small to be seen with the eye, but observed that it appeared to consist of a network of fine lines. In the 1970s a doctor in North Korea claimed to be able to demonstrate a network identical to that described by Sir Thomas; its fine threads are filled with a colorless transparent fluid. In an article in the Indian journal *Yoga-Mimansa*, the eminent Indian academic, Mat Rozmarynowski, wrote that in yoga, "the Nadis are said to be in the Pranic or astral body, because Prana, Nadis and the Chakras (the body's energy centers), are not visible to most people, only to yogis trained in Prana Vidya (the science of Prana) or to psychics."

When energy or prana flows from its reserve at the base of the spine, called kundalini, it rises through the central nadi, called sushumna, which passes through the spinal column. From the spinal column, it enters the skull and is experienced as an intense burst of energy. If this happens to someone who is unready for it, the experience can be devastating, so it must be permitted to happen only under controlled conditions, after a long and extremely careful process of preparation. One man who experienced the uncontrolled force of kundalini, an Indian, Gopi Krishna, subsequently devoted his life to experimenting with ways of releasing and controlling this energy, and wrote many books on his findings.

The twisting serpents represent the curved energy pathways, ida and pingala, entwined around the sushumna, the central nadi.

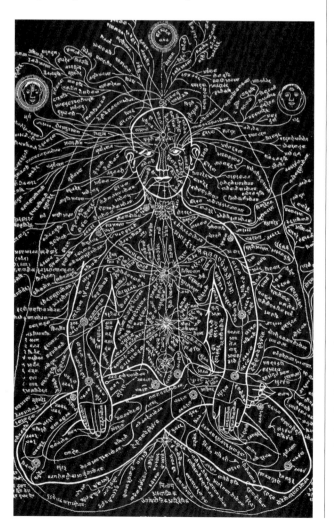

This illustration from an ancient yogic text depicts the body's energy system, the channels through which the life force, or prana, flows.

THE PRINCIPAL NADIS

Yoga teaches that a vast reserve of latent energy exists in every human being at the base of the spine. This energy is called kundalini, usually translated as "serpent power." It is claimed that three principal energy channels or nadis, rise from this point and end in the skull. The central channel, said to rise through the spinal column, is called sushumna; ida rises through the trunk and ends in the left nostril; and pingala ends in the right nostril. Ida and pingala are thought to crisscross as they rise, and the points at which they cross over are the sites of the chakras or wheels of energy.

CAUTION

Yoga asanas and breathing techniques aim at freeing the body's flow of energy in a controlled way. Most students who practice the asanas correctly and who persevere notice changes in their energy levels, and find they can increase their store of energy. But attempting to release kundalini energy is not something students should try without expert guidance.

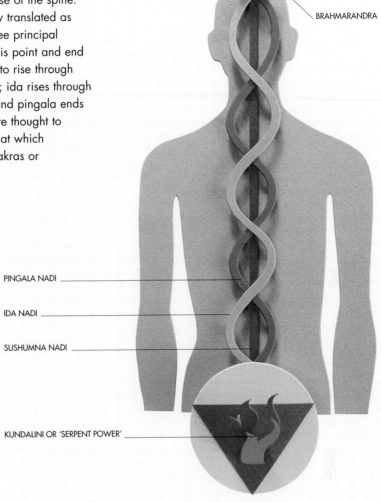

BRAHMARANDRA

PINGALA NADI

IDA NADI

SUSHUMNA NADI

KUNDALINI OR 'SERPENT POWER'

THE HEMISPHERES OF THE BRAIN

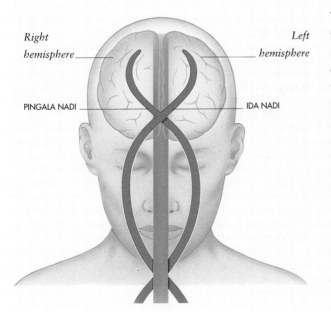

Right hemisphere

Left hemisphere

PINGALA NADI

IDA NADI

The body's energy rises from the base of the spine, from where it is channeled to the head along three main nadis. The flow of energy through two of these, called ida and pingala, is believed to relate directly to the functioning respectively of the right and left hemispheres of the brain. The right hemisphere is stimulated when we breathe through the left nostril, and vice versa. Recent medical research has shown that different mental functions are seated in different brain hemispheres – so singing and playing a musical instrument, for instance, are seated in the right hemisphere, while the ability to compose music is a left-hemisphere function. Not everyone is alike, however. In most people language ability is seated in the left hemisphere, but in some people it is in the right hemisphere and others have language-processing centers in both hemispheres.

The Body's Natural Design

An important principle of yoga is that it seeks to maintain the natural balance found in all aspects of life. The body's design incorporates a whole set of balances. Breathing, for example, maintains a balance between the body's demand for energy and the supply of oxygen to provide that energy. Yoga exercises sustain that balance by restoring the equilibrium between the breathing processes governed by the brain's physical-chemical feedback system, and those under our conscious control. To do this, yoga utilizes the body's natural design.

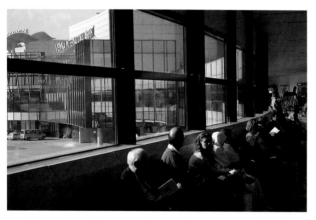

Poor posture increases the tension many people feel when traveling, especially by air.

Most people are dissatisfied with their body, if statistics are to be believed, and worry over what seem to be small deformities. But the apparent imperfections that create such anxiety are usually due to our own defective notions of a perfect body. Most people are born with a body whose purposeful design (see pages 22–23) has reached the pinnacle of perfection. Yet, by the time we have become adults, most have created distortions in the way their bodies work. Rather than try to narrow our hips or broaden our chests, we would benefit more from remedying some of the damage we have done imperceptibly over the years to our bones and muscles.

From the balance of the head to the pressure on the feet, the way people stand, walk, and sit affects their breathing. Poor posture is the most common cause of ineffective breathing and, consequently, of low energy levels, unhealthy muscular tension, and pessimistic or rigid outlook. Watch crowds at a rail terminus or an airport and it is clear that few people stand, walk, or sit with an erect posture. Most fall into two main physical types: those who slump, pigeon-chested, head poking forward, tensed up

or depressed; and those with thrust-out chest, permanently tensed abdominal muscles, and back-ward-leaning stance, seemingly challenging the world with their self-importance. It takes years to develop such ingrained habits of posture, and it is now generally accepted that their origins are rooted in childhood events and the stances adopted to deal with them.

Left uncorrected, these distorted stances damage the spine, the joints, the lungs, and the digestive system. With perseverence, however, yoga asanas will arrest such damage and gradually restore the body's system of balances. They will gently tighten unused, flaccid muscles, and restore movement to muscles made spastic through being held rigid, freeing the spinal bones into their natural positions, releasing pressure on the heart, the lungs, and the colon, and empowering the breathing to function naturally.

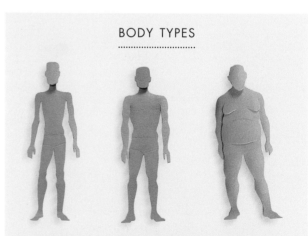

BODY TYPES

Whether you are slight, muscular, or heavily built makes no difference to your ability to do yoga – although a person with a large abdomen might find forward bends a struggle to achieve. Yoga changes the body from inside, making it more satisfyingly supple and more comfortable to live in.

AWARENESS OF THE BODY'S NATURAL STANCE

Yoga does not set out to alter natural life, but to enhance it. One of the main aims of the asanas is to enable the body to function as it was designed to work, and to correct the distortions caused over time by habitually standing, sitting, and walking in unnatural ways.

The balance of the head is naturally upright. Imagine a thread passing from the feet through the body and emerging from the crown of the head.

The collar bone should be in its natural position, not misaligned by abnormal carriage of the shoulders.

Correct head positioning ensures that no abnormal pressure is exerted on the muscles of the neck or the cervical vertebrae (neck) bones.

The shoulders should be comfortably balanced, not hunched up or pushed back.

The trunk held upright when sitting or standing counterbalances the natural curves of the spine.

The two curves of the spine are naturally accented when the trunk is held upright, but distorted when the back is held ramrod-straight, the trunk bent forward or the chest thrust out when standing or walking.

The stomach muscles naturally protrude slightly during out-breaths, but the stomach is held fairly flat by the proper tension of the stomach muscles.

The lower spine has a natural curve, so that the behind should protrude slightly. Trying to tuck it in distorts the spine and reduces the energy supply to the legs and feet.

The hips are held in their natural position when the trunk is upright. Thrusting them forward puts undue strain on the joints and thrusting them back depletes the supply of energy to the lower body.

When sitting the spine should be held upright. Allowing the weight to collapse onto the hips puts pressure on the hip joints.

Excessive body weight and distortions in the carriage of the upper body throw extra pressure on the knee joints.

Excessive body weight and distortions in the carriage of the upper body put undue pressure on the ankle joints and throw the balance out of alignment, resulting in an unnatural gait.

Correct Sitting

....

Mood sometimes results in poor posture in the upper body, because posture is a physical expression of a mental state. When people are depressed, they tend to slump; suddenly lifting the head and straightening the shoulders may feel like a false attempt to appear cheerful. Yet sitting upright does more than align the bones and muscles, it makes the breathing more effective because the passage of the air is not obstructed. This allows the diaphragm to move freely, improving circulation and stimulating the body's neuroelectrical system.

It can be difficult to judge whether one's own posture is good or needs some correction. The paper cup test illustrated opposite is a good way of finding out. Some people tend to sit, stand, and walk with their head and shoulders thrown right back, so a paper cup balanced on the crown of the head tends to slide off backward. The cup will slide forward from the head of anyone who habitually slumps. Anyone who has developed bad posture habits over a number of years needs to stretch the cramped muscles and retrain them over time. Exercise routines to do this are quite simple and extremely effective as long as they are carried out regularly.

Many of the asanas in the following chapters are performed sitting on the floor, on the heels or in one of the many cross-legged positions that have evolved over the centuries, so it is necessary to learn to sit in different ways. Good posture is the key, for it is impossible to perform the seated asanas correctly until correct sitting has become a way of life.

THE SPINE
....

The spine is not a straight column but an extraordinarily flexible structure of 33 small bones called vertebrae, which are cushioned by disks of cartilage and bound together by tough fibers called ligaments. The spine has two major curves: the cervical vertebrae curve forward and the thoracic vertebrae curve backward; while the lumbar section curves forward and the pelvic section backward. Attached to the vertebrae are several groups of muscles which control the spinal movements. The lumbar curve is more pronounced in women than in men, and the lumbar section of the spine is subjected to most pressure when posture is poor, especially when lifting heavy objects.

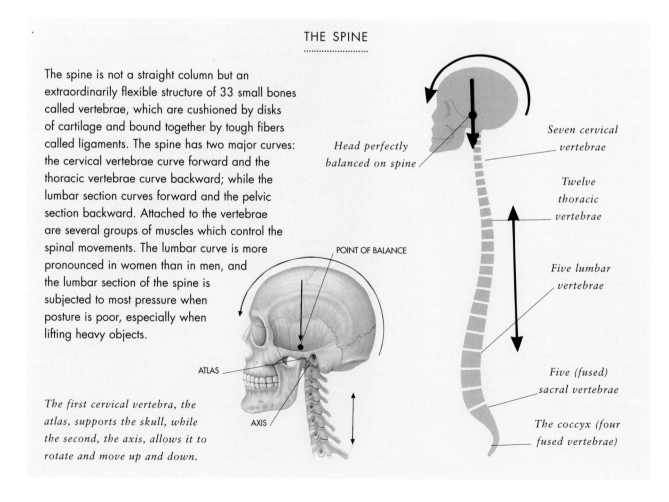

Head perfectly balanced on spine

Seven cervical vertebrae

Twelve thoracic vertebrae

Five lumbar vertebrae

Five (fused) sacral vertebrae

The coccyx (four fused vertebrae)

POINT OF BALANCE

ATLAS

AXIS

The first cervical vertebra, the atlas, supports the skull, while the second, the axis, allows it to rotate and move up and down.

SITTING ERECT

The body is designed to sit with the shoulders straight and the back, neck, and head upright. The opposing pulls of all the muscles balance out and align the bones correctly when the body is seated upright. This does not mean that you should strive to straighten your spine, however. The Victorian dame school tradition of strapping a board to children's backs to straighten the spine was very misguided – trying to sit bolt upright is unnatural because the spine has two curves. A well-designed chair can take a lot of hard work out of sitting correctly, so check that all chairs you sit on regularly are ergonomically designed. A poorly designed chair will quickly feel uncomfortable, and it is better to use your own muscle power to sit erect rather than slump against a badly shaped and positioned chair back.

THE PAPER CUP TEST

When seated working at a desk or a table, place a paper cup upside down on the crown of your head. At first it may fall off every few seconds, but as your posture improves it will stay on for a minute at a time, and gradually for longer. Once you can keep it in place for at least 5 minutes a bonus emerges: because the muscles remain flexible, there is no discomfort and breathing is unobstructed. Work becomes less tiring and concentration intensifies.

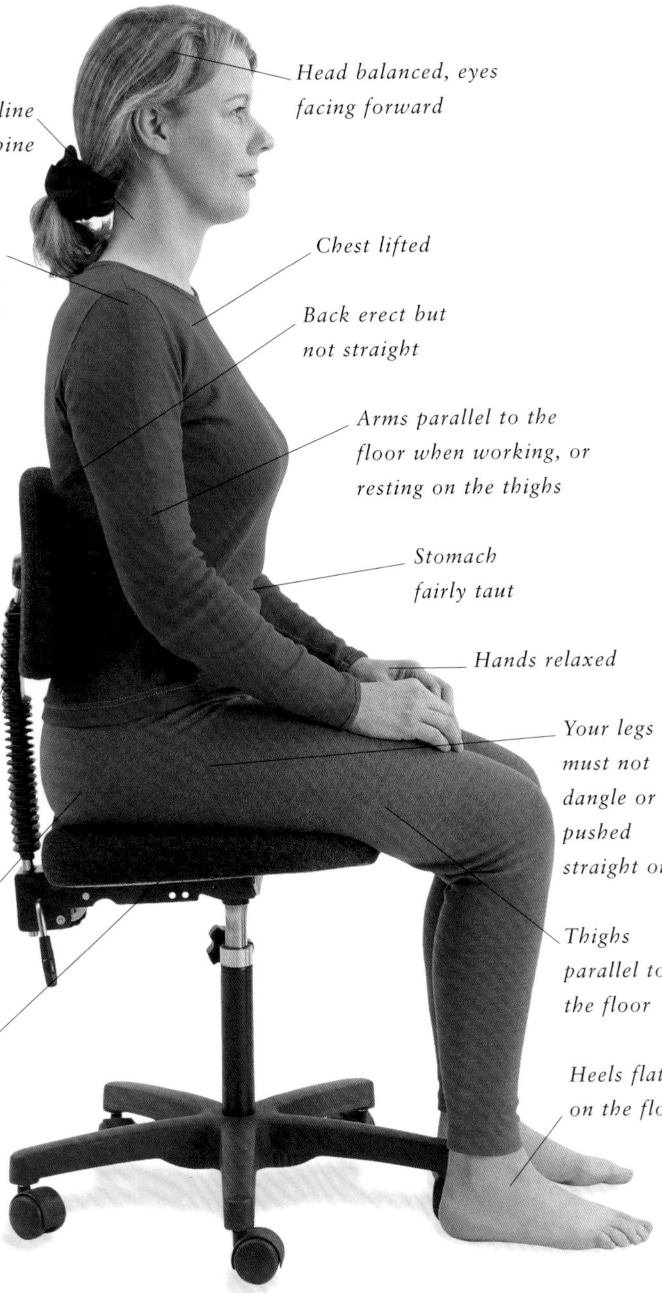

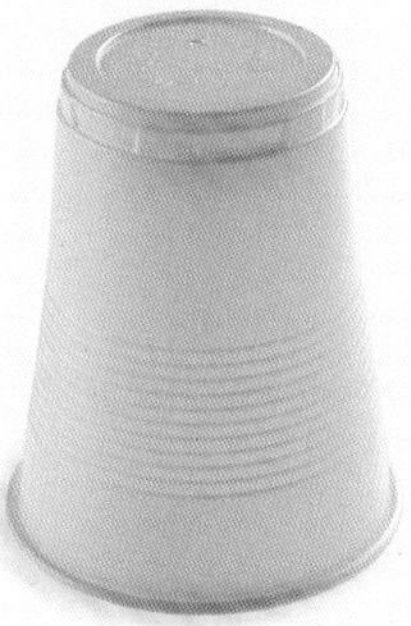

Neck in line with spine

Shoulders straight and relaxed

Head balanced, eyes facing forward

Chest lifted

Back erect but not straight

Arms parallel to the floor when working, or resting on the thighs

Stomach fairly taut

Hands relaxed

Your legs must not dangle or be pushed straight out

Thighs parallel to the floor

Heels flat on the floor

The chair back should be curved to support your spine.

Seat well back against the chair back

The front edge of the seat should curve downward. A straight edge gradually reduces the circulation in the legs.

The Body and Mind

Yoga is a holistic discipline and it teaches that nothing is wholly physical and nothing entirely mental. It emphasizes the unceasing interplay between mind and body. Anyone who has ever tried to change an ingrained habit knows how hard it is to reprogram the simplest reflex. Yoga techniques work on the interaction between mind and body to achieve changes on the physical and the mental level.

Yoga helps students alter their own awareness by gradually overriding some of the thousands of messages that flash every second between body and brain and replacing them with new sets of instructions. Repetition is the key. Learning about the benefits of good posture, stretching muscles that are underused or overworked, and spending time, day after day after day, consciously sitting in ways that benefit breathing will, in time, make the student more and more sensitive to the need for change and so help to bring the change about.

The way to success is not to expect miracles in a week or a month, but to work on raising awareness in the long term. Students must quiz themselves, often: Am I sitting up straight? Are my shoulders relaxed? They need to nag themselves: I'm going to work on my breathing at least four evenings this week. I always forget about the way I'm sitting when I'm with my friends. It is always a surprise to those who persevere to discover suddenly that the goalposts are way behind, to catch sight of themselves in a mirror and realize that they are now sitting erect without having to remind themselves. Things have changed and it is time to move on to tackle new aims, new ways of sitting, and new asanas.

WATCHING OTHERS

The way people stand and sit when they are waiting, walking, and hurrying reveals that few people maintain erect carriage, and their body posture tells you a great deal about their inner life. Quietly observing other people is an excellent way of raising your own consciousness of the way the body and mind work together, and can help you overcome obstacles to your own progress toward efficient, beneficial sitting and standing.

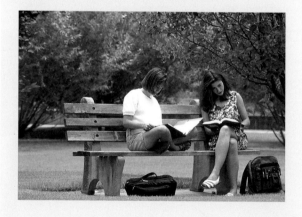

DRIVING

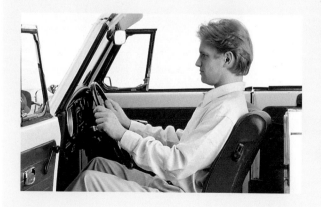

People tend to forget all about posture when they are driving, yet poor attention to posture affects the two factors that are essential to safe driving: concentration and self-control. Maintaining control over the body ensures efficient breathing and keeps your concentration active, enabling you to assess new situations accurately and to react to them quickly. It also helps you keep dangerous emotions, such as impatience, in check, preventing them from exploding into rage.

THE NERVOUS SYSTEM

Some 200,000 messages a minute travel between the brain and the nervous system. Receptors inside the body and on its surface transmit reports on changes in local conditions in the form of electrical impulses, which travel along the motor fibers in the nerves to the brain. In the brain's receptor centers the signals are interpreted and impulses sent along the sensory fibers in the nerves to muscles, for example, ordering them to move or rest, or to glands, ordering them to become active or stop secreting. The speed of electrical impulses carrying such messages is measured in milliseconds.

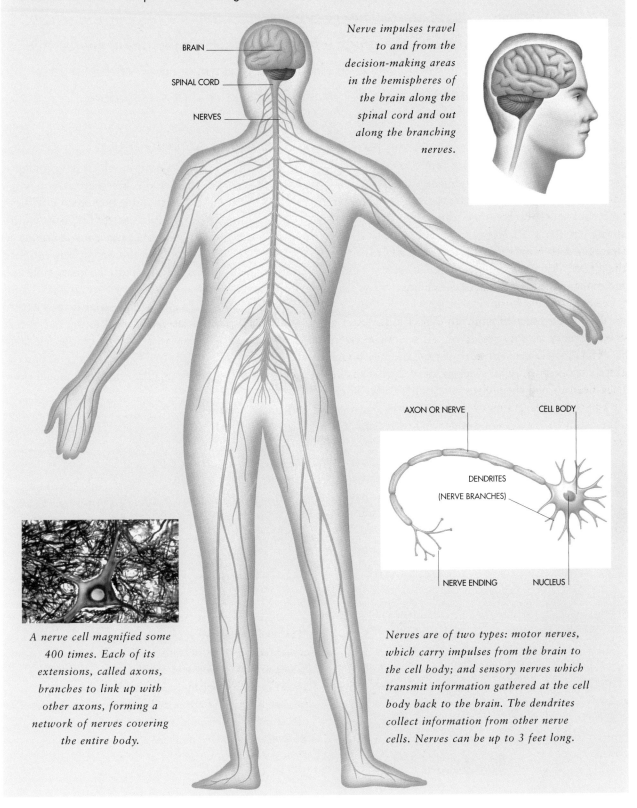

BRAIN

SPINAL CORD

NERVES

Nerve impulses travel to and from the decision-making areas in the hemispheres of the brain along the spinal cord and out along the branching nerves.

AXON OR NERVE

CELL BODY

DENDRITES
(NERVE BRANCHES)

NERVE ENDING

NUCLEUS

A nerve cell magnified some 400 times. Each of its extensions, called axons, branches to link up with other axons, forming a network of nerves covering the entire body.

Nerves are of two types: motor nerves, which carry impulses from the brain to the cell body; and sensory nerves which transmit information gathered at the cell body back to the brain. The dendrites collect information from other nerve cells. Nerves can be up to 3 feet long.

Pelvic Flexibility

Many of the yoga asanas are performed sitting on the floor, and there are numerous conflicting opinions about the best way to sit in order to perform them. Some people, especially children, whose joints and muscles are very flexible, sit naturally in almost any position – including the full lotus in which each foot rests on the opposite thigh – but most older people find it impossible to sit cross-legged for any length of time. It can be more comfortable at first to kneel, Japanese-style, for breathing practice and meditation.

Sitting cross-legged can be uncomfortable for anyone whose muscles and joints are stiff through lack of exercise and many students need to spend time on exercise, to improve their flexibility before they can adapt to sitting on the floor. Beginners may prefer simply to kneel on the floor and sit back on the heels. The muscles stretch quickly, however, and as long as the back is erect, it is soon possible to sit cross-legged for as long as an hour without any discomfort or circulatory problems.

The cross-legged position most closely associated with yoga is the

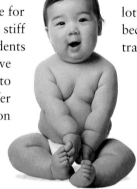

Yoga enables adults to regain some of the pelvic flexibility they had as young children.

lotus position. Many students want to do this because it is a position in which the Buddha is traditionally depicted – but there is no special virtue in doing it. Some people do it without any effort, but other people find it very difficult and need to spend time learning it. Attempting to do it the wrong way can load damaging stress onto the knee joint, so it is not a good idea to try to teach yourself. As always, the goal here is not to show off what you can do, but to find a position in which you can sit comfortably for long enough to practice breathing, relaxation, and meditation.

SITTING ON THE HEELS

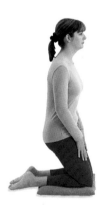

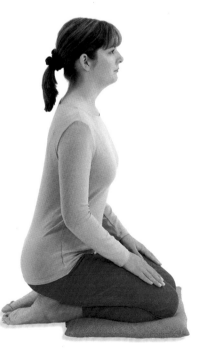

The simplest way of sitting on the floor is to sit back on the heels, Japanese-style. If your body is somewhat stiff overall, perhaps because of lack of exercise, you will find this beneficial because it stretches the long quadriceps muscles at the front of the thighs, which straighten the knees.

1 *Kneel on a cushion at first. Lower yourself onto your knees gently in order not to damage the quadriceps by abrupt stretching.*

2 *Now sit back on your heels. Sit up, straighten the shoulders, and check that your head is erect. Then rest your hands on your thighs. At first you may be able to sit on the heels for only a few minutes. Practice regularly, keeping a straight back and do not permit yourself to sink down onto your heels, and you will be able to sit for longer and longer periods.*

CROSS-LEGGED SITTING

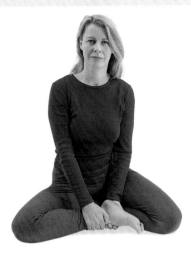

This exercise is designed to make the thigh joints and the tendons and muscles of the legs more flexible. You may be able to manage only the first four steps at first. Treat the thigh muscles and the knee joints firmly – but gently. Trying to force them to do too much too quickly might damage them.

1 *Sit in a simple cross-legged position on a mat, with the right ankle crossing over the left. Check that your posture is erect. Push your left heel as far into your groin as you can.*

2 *Lift your right ankle, using both hands, while using your leg muscles to pull the right knee down. Repeat the exercise ten times, making a rhythmic movement.*

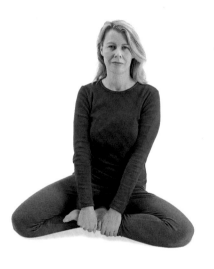

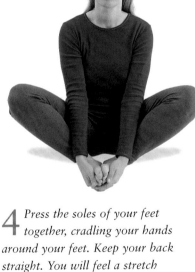

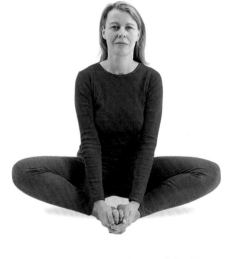

3 *Repeat steps 1 and 2 with the opposite leg. Then rest your hands on your knees.*

4 *Press the soles of your feet together, cradling your hands around your feet. Keep your back straight. You will feel a stretch across the groin.*

5 *Still holding your feet with both hands, move your knees up and down. This is called the butterfly movement and it should be performed rhythmically. You may feel strain across the groin, but try to keep up the rhythm for two to three minutes and the muscles should stretch, easing the strained feeling.*

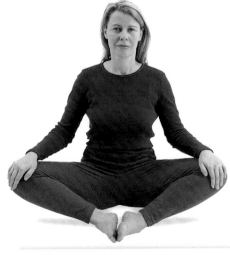

6 *Keep the soles of the feet pressed together, put one hand on each knee and gently press down.*

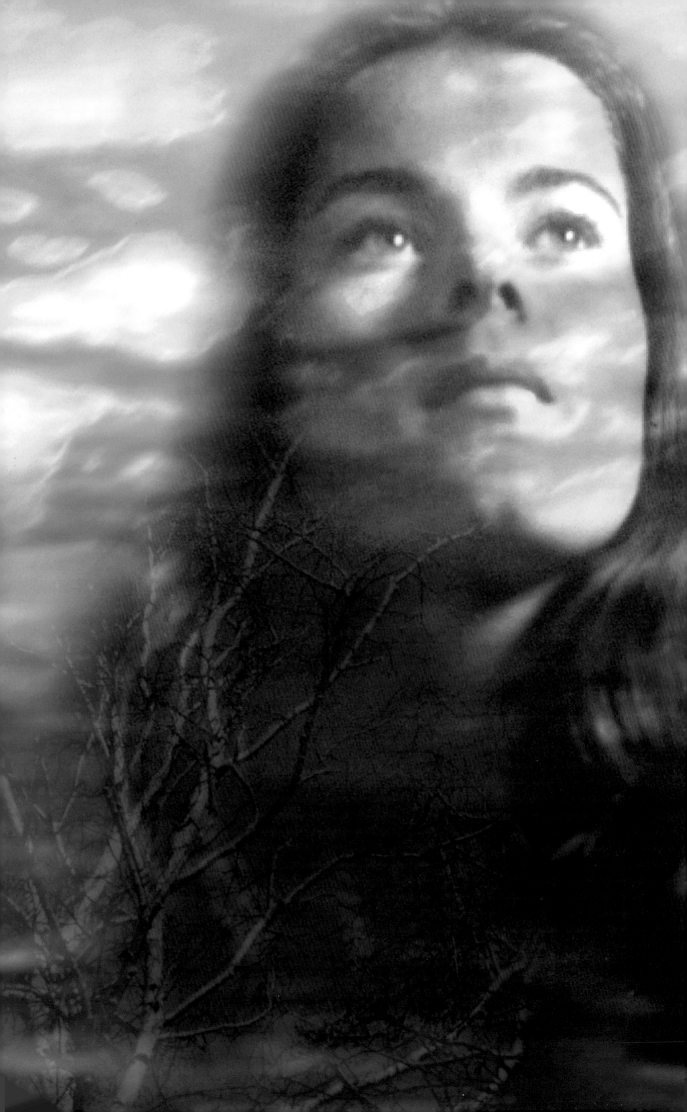

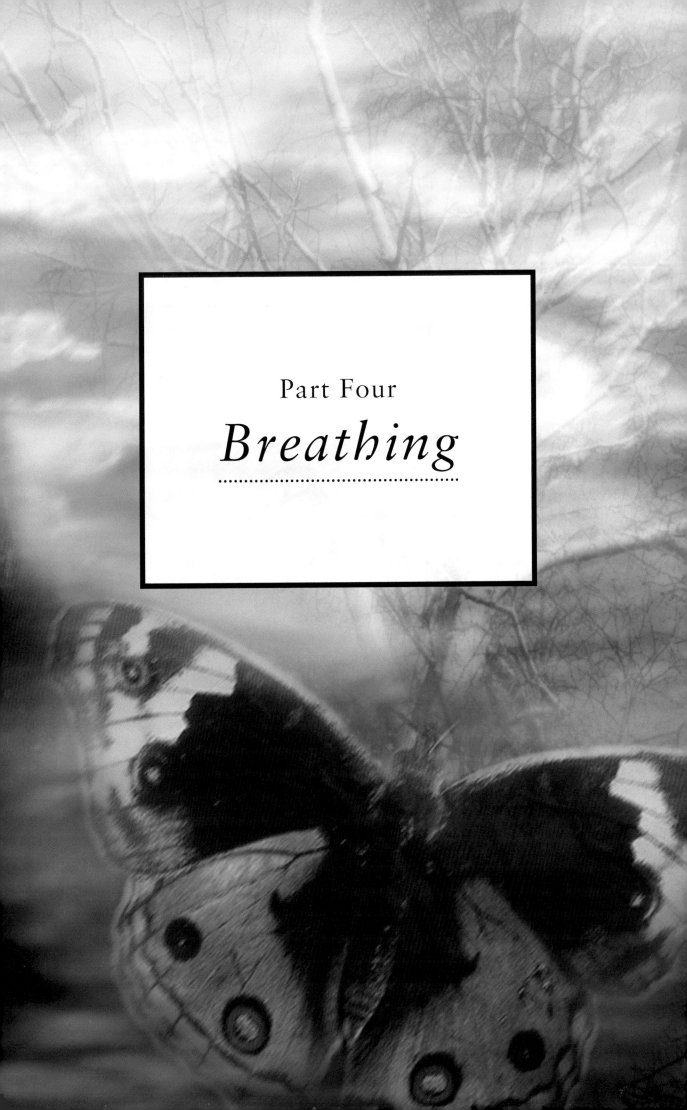

Part Four
Breathing

Importance of Breathing

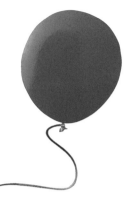

Effective breathing is the key to the practice of yoga. The timing of an out-breath can make it possible to stretch a little further, or to finally master a difficult asana. Without correct breathing true relaxation is impossible and peace of mind is hard to achieve. Poor breathing affects the body in other ways, sapping the energy, undermining the immune system, making the body more prone to illness, and making us irritable.

The impulse to breathe is involuntary, controlled by the respiratory center in the brain-stem, so that we breathe when we are babies, when we sleep, and when we are not concentrating on breathing. Very early in life, however, the depth and rate of breathing are brought under voluntary control, and they are governed to a large degree by the state of the emotions. We are all instinctively aware that fear, sorrow, depression, and high excitement inhibit the intake of breath – writers speak of people catching their breath in alarm or elation, make a threatening character breathe heavily, and a victim sigh with relief when a threat has passed.

There may be good physical reasons for the evolution of the emotional control of breathing. Angry people pant – to speed the flow of blood to the muscles, in case they need to fight. A person experiencing a sudden, sharp pain might stop breathing momentarily – to reduce the intensity of feeling until the spasm has passed. In normal life, breathing is not often called upon to deal with such emotional emergencies, yet as every yoga teacher knows, most people, when tested, find it difficult to breathe naturally. The

blame for this can often be traced to individuals' responses to stresses and strains in their life. An unloved child, for instance, may resort to permanent shallow breathing to deaden the pain of neglect, while panting may become a way of life for a person whose anger has become habitual.

For almost everyone a large part of learning yoga must therefore involve understanding their own breathing pattern, unlearning it, and slowly learning to breathe again in a different way. The process can be difficult, for it can take weeks to assimilate new breathing habits, but perseverance pays. Correct breathing not only makes it easier to stretch and execute the asanas correctly, it brings other, astonishing rewards. Breathing correctly strengthens not just the muscles but all the body's internal systems. Good breathing neutralizes the daily effects of stress and improves health by reducing blood pressure, improving the circulation, and strengthening the neuro-electrical system. It boosts the immune system, preventing illness. And controlled breathing is the fastest and most effective way of breaking down anxiety and anger and lifting depression. An individual who breathes better will also feel better from head to toe, inside and out.

You should bear in mind that a relaxed, erect posture is the key to good breathing habits. It is equally important to develop the habit of breathing through the nose and not through the mouth. Air is warmed as it passes from the nose into the lungs, and minute, mucus-covered hairs in the nostrils trap particles which might damage the lungs.

The following pages explain how breathing works and show how to recognize damaging breathing habits that may have developed over many years. They illustrate how to unlearn unnatural breathing and how to learn new ways of breathing to create energy and ensure true relaxation.

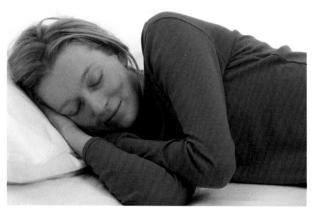

Effective breathing relaxes body and mind, making it easier to slip into a good night's sleep.

HOW TO BREATHE

The diaphragm is a large muscle that separates the chest from the abdomen. To draw inhaled air from the nose into the lungs, the muscle fibers of the diaphragm and the intercostal muscles (thin sheets of muscle between the lower ribs) all contract. This expands the chest, and air is drawn into the lungs to fill the space.

During normal breathing the trunk (the chest and abdomen) acts as a pump. As you breathe in you tense the abdominal muscles slightly, and as you exhale you release them. This causes a squeeze-release effect in the abdomen: the downward movement of the diaphragm and the tension in the abdominal wall reduces the space in the abdomen, so the organs inside it are squeezed or "massaged" and their blood supply increases. This abdominal massaging benefits digestion and helps to prevent disorders such as irritable bowel syndrome.

INHALING

EXHALING

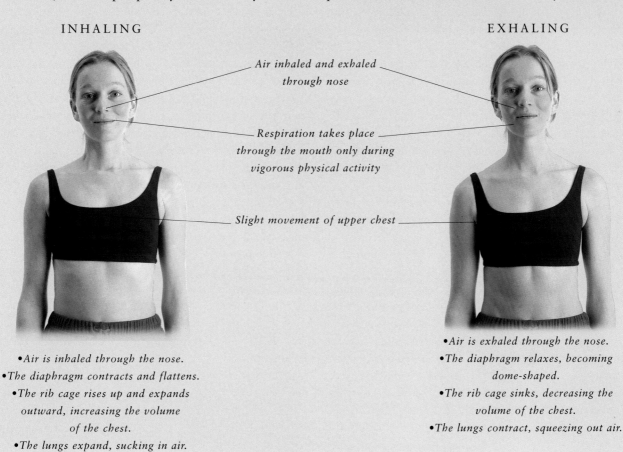

Air inhaled and exhaled through nose

Respiration takes place through the mouth only during vigorous physical activity

Slight movement of upper chest

- *Air is inhaled through the nose.*
- *The diaphragm contracts and flattens.*
- *The rib cage rises up and expands outward, increasing the volume of the chest.*
- *The lungs expand, sucking in air.*

- *Air is exhaled through the nose.*
- *The diaphragm relaxes, becoming dome-shaped.*
- *The rib cage sinks, decreasing the volume of the chest.*
- *The lungs contract, squeezing out air.*

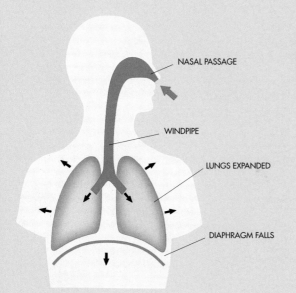

NASAL PASSAGE

WINDPIPE

LUNGS EXPANDED

DIAPHRAGM FALLS

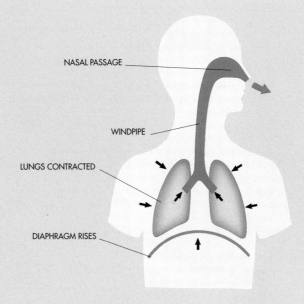

NASAL PASSAGE

WINDPIPE

LUNGS CONTRACTED

DIAPHRAGM RISES

Learning to Breathe

A person who breathes naturally breathes in a relaxed, rhythmical way, neither very deeply nor very shallowly. For many people, trying to breathe in this way is so difficult that it makes them realize how bad their breathing has become.

Practicing the art of breathing involves learning once again to use the muscles that control breathing. For example, people who are tense find it hard to breathe out and have to practice relaxing the muscles of the ribs and abdomen. Physicians in the West have tended to overlook the contribution that natural breathing can make to health, which may be why shallow breathing is one of the most common problems in Western societies. An important function of breathing is to maintain the balance of oxygen to carbon dioxide in the blood, and if this balance is disrupted, faintness and numbness can result.

Yogis believe that breathing techniques taught in the West may be based on certain wrong assumptions.

For instance, breathing exercises often begin with a deep in-breath, but yoga teaches that good respiration begins with a long, slow exhalation. The lungs never empty completely during exhalation, nor do they fill completely during inhalation; the air breathed in mixes with the 10 percent of stale air that always remains in the lungs to keep them inflated. Instead, the aim is to breathe out as completely as possible, so that on the next in-breath the greatest amount of fresh air is breathed in to vitalize the body.

Breathing correctly is essential to life, to health, and to effective yoga, so that it is important to practice breathing at least once a day for three months or longer, until effective breathing has become natural.

SHALLOW BREATHING

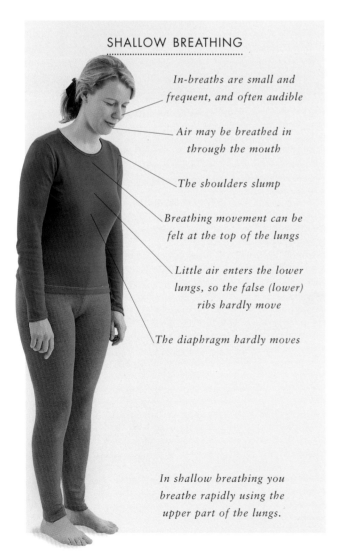

In-breaths are small and frequent, and often audible

Air may be breathed in through the mouth

The shoulders slump

Breathing movement can be felt at the top of the lungs

Little air enters the lower lungs, so the false (lower) ribs hardly move

The diaphragm hardly moves

In shallow breathing you breathe rapidly using the upper part of the lungs.

TENSE BREATHING

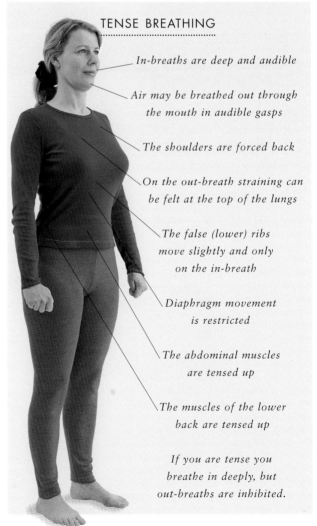

In-breaths are deep and audible

Air may be breathed out through the mouth in audible gasps

The shoulders are forced back

On the out-breath straining can be felt at the top of the lungs

The false (lower) ribs move slightly and only on the in-breath

Diaphragm movement is restricted

The abdominal muscles are tensed up

The muscles of the lower back are tensed up

If you are tense you breathe in deeply, but out-breaths are inhibited.

TESTING YOUR BREATHING

*You can do this exercise even if you are unused
to deep breathing, or if you are stiff. You can sit
on a chair or lie on the floor.*

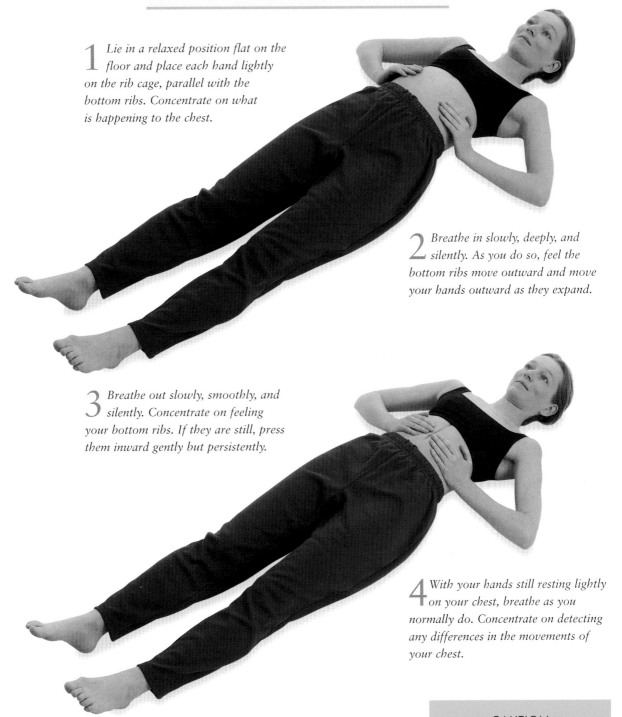

1 *Lie in a relaxed position flat on the
floor and place each hand lightly
on the rib cage, parallel with the
bottom ribs. Concentrate on what
is happening to the chest.*

2 *Breathe in slowly, deeply, and
silently. As you do so, feel the
bottom ribs move outward and move
your hands outward as they expand.*

3 *Breathe out slowly, smoothly, and
silently. Concentrate on feeling
your bottom ribs. If they are still, press
them inward gently but persistently.*

4 *With your hands still resting lightly
on your chest, breathe as you
normally do. Concentrate on detecting
any differences in the movements of
your chest.*

5 *Repeat steps 1–3, squeezing the
ribs on out-breaths and releasing
on in-breaths, for up to five minutes.
Relax for a few minutes before
getting up.*

CAUTION

If your ribs have recently been
broken or bruised, or your chest
has been damaged, do not
attempt this exercise.

Breathing for Energy and Relaxation

Learning to breathe naturally has two immediate benefits that are much in demand in the modern world: it spirits away fatigue and revivifies mind and body. Natural breathing can marshall frazzled nerves into a state of relaxation in a very short time, and it is a magic wand that fades out exhaustion and replaces it with energy, plucked – literally – from thin air.

Breathing is essentially an automatic process, though under the control of the brain. Although a surprising amount of voluntary activity controls this vital bodily function, interfering with the breathing can have unexpected effects. If, for example, we try to change our breathing pattern by slowing it down, in order to be able to relax, the mere fact of trying to impose willpower on the breathing causes conflict, which impedes relaxation. Yoga teaches ways of arousing awareness of the body, the role breathing plays in its functioning, and the physical and mental differences between tension and relaxation. Little by little, as students practice exercises and asanas, they become gradually more aware of abnormalities in breathing, of how their physical and mental tensions affect their breathing, and of how the way they breathe affects their bodies and minds. Without directly seeking to change their breathing, the students' breathing patterns gradually modify themselves.

In the 1970s Britain's leading medical journal, the *Lancet*, carried two reports by a hospital doctor, Chandra Patel, of experiments she carried out on helping people with hypertension – high blood pressure. In controlled trials she produced remarkable results in a range of patients, some of whom had been on medication for up to 17 years. Dr Patel found that a yoga relaxation course improved the condition in almost all participants, some losing all their symtoms. These effects were subsequently found to be lasting.

CHANGING YOUR BREATHING RATE

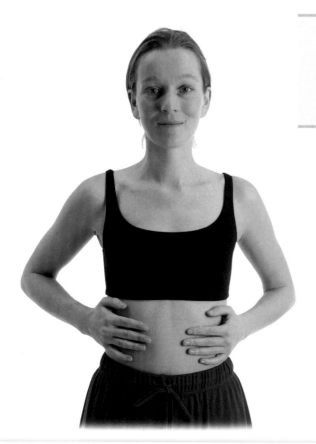

This exercise shows how easy it is to change your rate of breathing temporarily. Anyone in moderate health can speed or slow their breathing, but it takes many practice sessions to change your breathing permanently, especially if you have developed unnatural breathing habits.

1 *Sit or stand where you can see a clock. Put your hands on your lower ribs and count the number of times you breathe in and out in one minute. The average person breathes 14 to 16 times in a minute.*

2 *Breathe faster and count the breaths (in and out) you take in one minute. You can speed your breathing without difficulty – after vigorous exercise you may take up to 80 breaths a minute.*

3 *Take a break, calm your breathing, then repeat the exercise, this time trying to breathe much more slowly than you normally do. With practice, breathing can be slowed to as few as six breaths a minute – the usual rate during meditation.*

INSTANT ENERGY

If you have a sedentary job or if you work at home, doing these exercises after work will make you feel energized. They stimulate the heart and circulation.

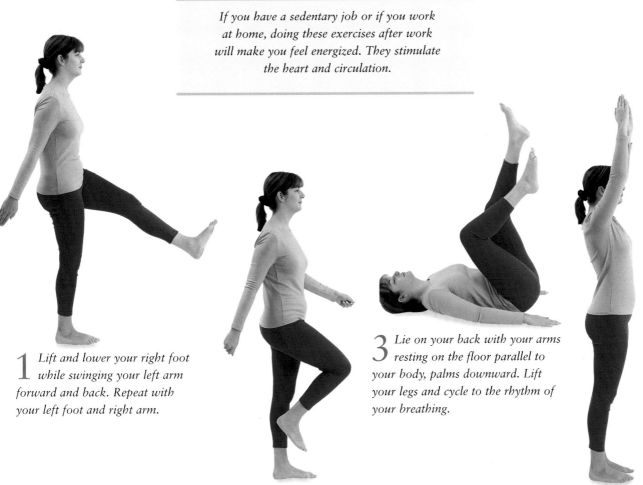

1 *Lift and lower your right foot while swinging your left arm forward and back. Repeat with your left foot and right arm.*

2 *March on the spot, then around the room or outdoors, always stepping with one leg while swinging the other arm, for about 5 minutes.*

3 *Lie on your back with your arms resting on the floor parallel to your body, palms downward. Lift your legs and cycle to the rhythm of your breathing.*

4 *Stand erect and, keeping your knees slightly bent, breathe in and swing your arms high up above your head, then let them fall as you breathe out. Repeat this exercise two or three times to stretch your trunk and arms.*

INSTANT RELAXATION

Being able to relax during the day is a valuable tool for dealing with continuous rush and stress, or prolonging concentration for effective study. There is no need to lie down, it is just as easy to relax sitting in a chair at the kitchen table, at a desk in an office or a library, or on a train. Sit upright for a few minutes with your hands resting on your lap, and concentrate on breathing slowly and effectively. Think about each part of your body in turn, consciously relaxing any muscles that seem tense. Let your mind go free.

Do not worry that you will forget the time or fall asleep. When you relax thoroughly, part of your mind remains aware of what is going on while your body is resting. At the end of the allotted time – 5 minutes, perhaps, or 15 – you will begin to feel alert. But the rest will have revived your body and cleared your mind of preoccupation with what was happening before. It releases your mind into a state from which it can move on and start concentrating effectively once again.

57

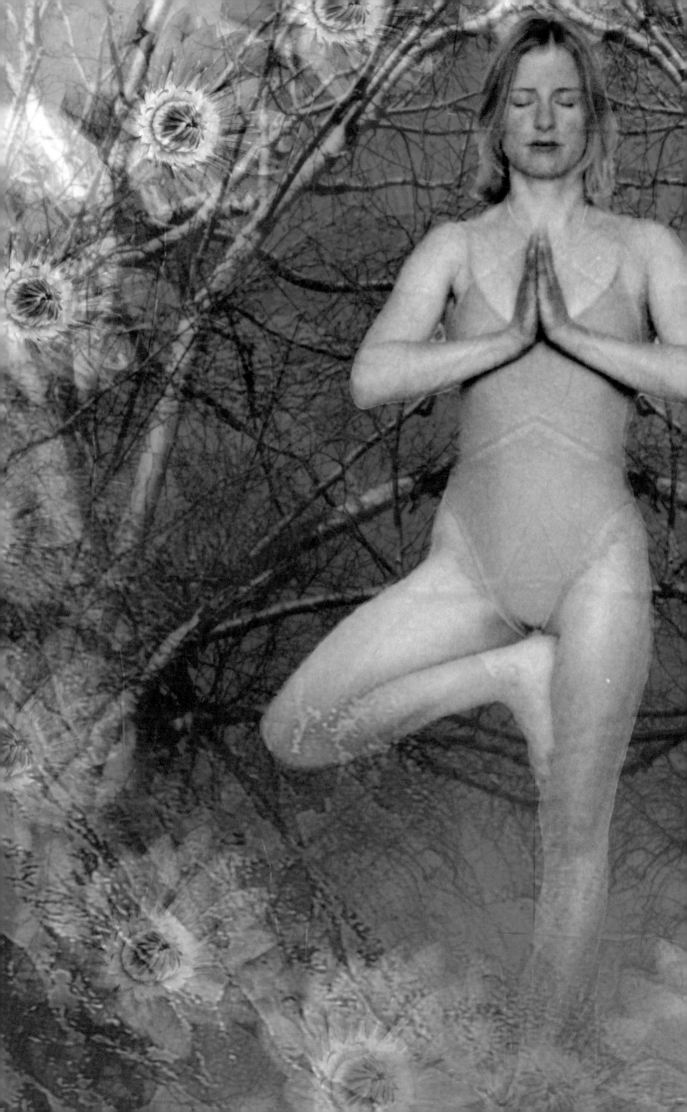

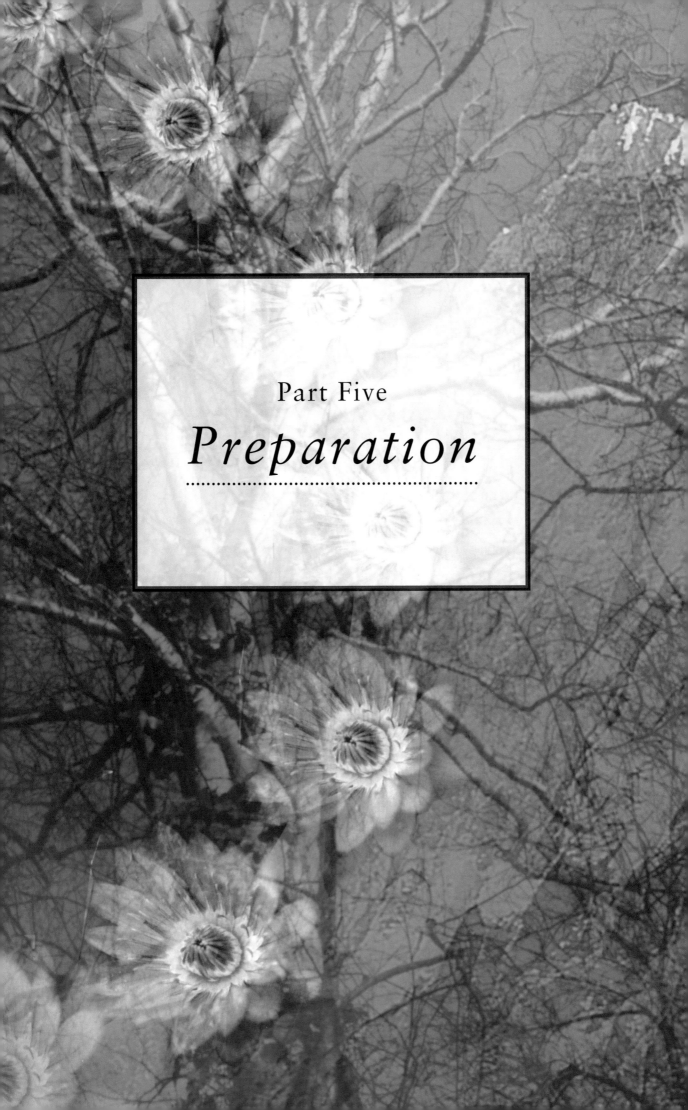

Part Five

Preparation

Planning a Yoga Program

In some ways the idea of planning a yoga program runs against the thinking behind yoga practice. Everyone's physiology and psychology are different, and the aim of yoga is to learn to listen to the body's own needs and to do what it wants to do. However, while some people work effectively in an unstructured way, others need to follow a set program, especially when they are beginning.

Before planning their program, all students should sit and think carefully about why they want to take up yoga and what they want to achieve. It is important to be realistic from the start: however enthusiastically you practice, yoga may never give you a more shapely body or make you lose weight. Focus on the idea that the main objective of yoga is to bring inner peace and harmony (see pages 18–19).

Yoga can fit very comfortably into different lifestyles. There is no ideal time of day to practice – yogis traditionally practice asanas for most of the day. Individual lifestyle dictates the time of day the sessions take place. There is only one rule: to be effective, practice must be regular – once a week at least, preferably three or four times a week, ideally once a day. There is no set duration for a class. The planner illustrated opposite allocates time for a 90-minute class, since 90 minutes is an optimum timespan for the human body (see pages 26–27), but it is possible to benefit from daily sessions lasting for 20–30 minutes each, or sessions that vary in duration from day to day and increase over time.

There are certain elements that every yoga program needs. Each session should begin with a few stretches and a moment of stillness, plus a few minutes of relaxation through breathing. Time working on the asanas needs to be punctuated by brief relaxation breaks. The session should end with breathing practice and several minutes of full relaxation.

Follow a backward bend with one that flexes the spine in the opposite direction.

Many yoga manuals suggest that the asanas should be practiced in a certain order based on the progressive exercising of different parts of the body. These considerations are not important, however. The asanas in this book may be practiced in almost any order, with the one proviso that it is essential to observe the principle of balance and counterbalance – a forward bend needs to be followed by a backward bend, and so on (see pages 82–83).

It may be helpful to keep notes on your progress.

At first, students often find they want to work on the back. This is to be highly recommended since greater flexibility in the spine makes it easier to master asanas affecting other parts of the body. Others might want to work on a stiff shoulder or on their hands and arms. It is perfectly possible to work on the back in one session and the hands, arms, and shoulders in another, and to plan short sessions for practicing balance or breathing. What is important in establishing a yoga program is to keep the whole picture in mind so that no part of the body is ignored.

Making progress means that the program will need to be replanned at intervals. Beginners may prefer to concentrate on exercise and breathing at the beginning and only try meditation and visualization (see pages 126–29) when they feel more confident.

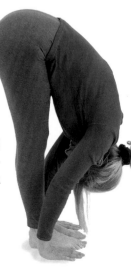

A forward bend counterbalances the effect of a backward bend.

ESSENTIAL ELEMENTS OF A PROGRAM

Objective: To improve the quality of my life.

Although yoga is partly physical, the exercise is merely a means to attain the mental calm needed for meditation. Beware of the mindset that idealizes physical perfection. In yoga the body does not always "improve" from an aesthetic point of view. But if you allow yoga to bring you inner happiness you may find your appearance changes.

1 **Warm-up stretches – 10 minutes:** *These relax the muscles and joints, warm the body, and speed the circulation ready for practice. Stretching banishes the stresses and excitements of the day, clears the mind, and focuses on the yoga session.*

2 **Relaxation – 1 minute:** *Always rest the muscles and joints for a short time after using them. Allow the mind to clear and focus on the next phase of action.*

3 **Breathing – 10 minutes:** *This cools off the body after vigorous exercise, slows the heartbeat, and induces greater flexibility. Breathing calms the thoughts, sharpens receptivity, and provides a pause for listening to the body and gauging what it wants.*

4 **Asanas sequence – 50 minutes:** *The sequence improves mobility, flexibility, and muscle control. It trains the mind in concentration and control of thoughts and emotions.*

5 **Breath Control – 10 minutes:** *This energizes the body's neuro-electrical system and generates a state of calm.*

6 **Full relaxation – 10 minutes:** *Allow the body to rest totally after exercise, and let the mind clear, ready for the next phase of action.*

SUGGESTED ASANA SEQUENCE	
ACTION	TIME
Half lotus	5 minutes
Cat and Dog	10 minutes
Pause to rest	1 minute
Spinal twist	10 minutes
Pause to rest	1 minute
Triangle and reverse triangle	5 minutes
Pause to rest	1 minute
Bow	5 minutes
Boat	5 minutes
Pause to rest	1 minute
Half candle	5 minutes

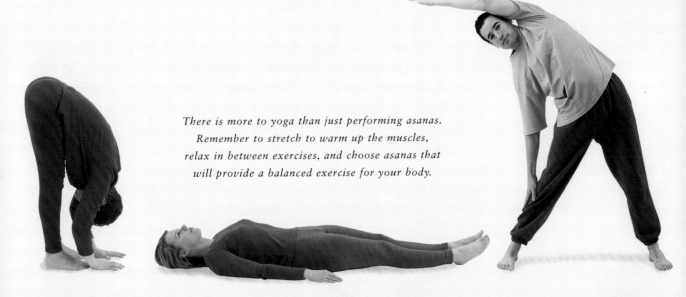

There is more to yoga than just performing asanas. Remember to stretch to warm up the muscles, relax in between exercises, and choose asanas that will provide a balanced exercise for your body.

Ensuring a Balanced Approach

Because yoga is a holistic discipline, balance is a central principle. In yoga sessions, time is allocated in equal proportion to asanas, breathing, relaxation, and, as expertise develops, to meditation, so that the body, the brain, and the mind are accorded equal importance.

The asanas are chosen to complement each other, obeying the principle of balance and counterbalance. The muscles work mainly in groups rather than individually, so that an asana that stretches and exercises one muscle group is always followed by one that works on another, complementary group. The exercises and asanas described in this book are all selected in accordance with this principle. So, for instance, the asana called the bridge, which bends the spine backward and stretches the muscles of the chest and abdomen, is followed by the boat, which bends the spine forward and tenses the abdominal muscles.

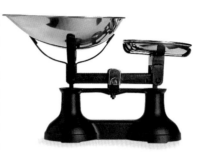

Yoga encourages moderation, calm, and a sense of proportion.

Yoga also gently teaches the art of forging a balance between work and relaxation. The muscles are tensed and stressed up to a certain point only. Once the movement becomes strained or painful it is stopped. A yoga session is punctuated by regular pauses for rest and relaxation, so that negative influences are eliminated. Yoga asanas, however difficult, never tire the body or mind. Instead, they invigorate.

Breathing maintains the balance between body and mind, and hatha yoga attaches much importance to learning to breathe correctly. Breathing relaxes the body and makes the mind receptive to meditation.

Applying the principle of balance in practice sessions is training for applying it in everyday life. As control of muscular tension and breathing become second nature, students find their whole philosophy of life changes. People nowadays often depend for happiness on exciting times to brighten their lives, feeling depressed and dissatisfied when situations fail to live up to their expectations. Yoga teaches people to find the source of happiness and satisfaction within themselves, and to regard the good times as unexpected bonuses in life, to be used as sources of inner strength. The idea is to enjoy happy events, to live them to the full as long as they last, but not to depend for enjoyment of life or peace of mind on their frequent recurrence. Instead, everyone needs to learn to live for the moment, drawing strength from the pleasurable events so that every moment is lived and enjoyed to its fullest extent. The result is that good times can be enjoyed without being marred by shadowy doubts that perhaps they should be even better.

YOGA VS. SPORT

An important difference between sports, such as golf, and yoga is that the same set of muscles needs to be used over and over again to achieve certain movements in many sports, while yoga ensures that using a set of muscles to achieve one particular movement, such as a spinal twist, is immediately balanced by a movement in the opposite direction which exercises the opposing muscle group. Yoga can therefore assist athletes by exercising their underused muscles. With this increased overall mobility and flexibility yoga can make a difference to sports performance.

Golfing uses a sequence of repetitive actions.

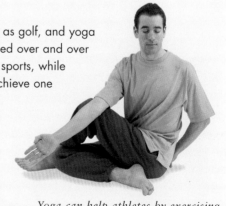

Yoga can help athletes by exercising underused muscle groups.

BALANCING THE BODY

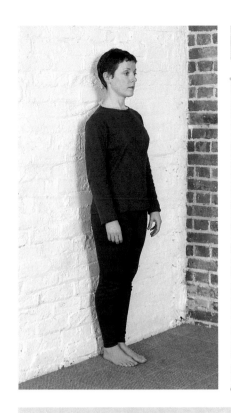

The art of balancing the body is paramount in yoga, and importance is given to learning to stand erect without leaning slightly backward or forward. Use the method illustrated here to check whether your posture is as upright as you assume it is. If the results reveal a tendency to lean, remind yourself to try to balance upright several times a day. Repeat the test regularly, even when you have trained your balance, since illness, injury, weight changes, and changes in the body resulting from aging and pregnancy can throw the body off balance.

1 Stand against a wall, with your heels half an inch away from it. Stand erect, then measure the distance between your head and the wall. If necessary, adjust your posture so that the back of your head is the same distance from the wall as your heels. Pause and try to remember how it feels to stand in that position.

2 Walk around the room, then return and try to stand with your heels and your head half an inch away from the wall. Measure the distance again. Repeat the exercise as often as necessary until your stance becomes truly upright.

TREE

Few people can stand for any length of time on one leg. The tree posture trains the sense of balance.

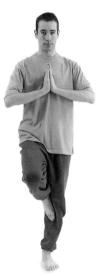

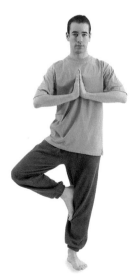

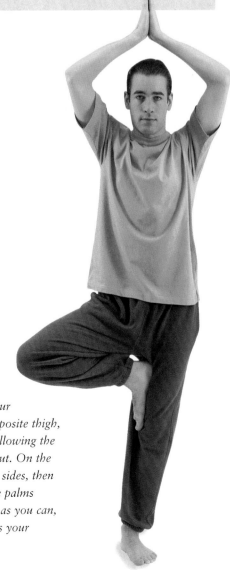

1 Stand erect with your hands by your sides. Rest one foot against the opposite knee and allow the bent knee to move backward and outward. Raise your hands to your chest in the namaste (prayer) position and close your eyes. Hold for as long as you can. Repeat with the other leg.

2 Stand erect with your hands by your sides. Rest one foot against the opposite thigh, pressing the heel into your groin and allowing the bent knee to move outward. Breathe out. On the in-breath, stretch your arms out to the sides, then lift them above your head, pressing the palms together. Hold your breath for as long as you can, then slowly lower your arms and leg as your breathe out. Repeat with the other leg.

Preparing for Yoga Practice

For yoga practice to be effective, the body needs to be flexible and the mind free. At the start of a session, however, there may be tensions in body and mind, so preparation is an important part of training. There is no set program to follow. The aim is simply to become more receptive.

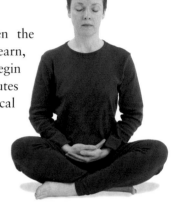

Relaxed breathing is a good way to cool off and calm down. The heartbeat will slow down and the sense of pressure will dissipate. Working the muscles stimulates the circulation and dispels lethargy, and simple stretching is a good way of warming up before starting work on the asanas.

The body must always be treated gently, with love. It is all too easy to begin by having a go at a new asana, but without preparation this could cause injury. That is why, no matter how pressurized the day has been or how keen the student may be to learn, practice must never begin without those few minutes of mental and physical preparation.

A degree of mental calmness will allow tense muscles to relax.

MOUNTAIN

Variation: *This variation on the mountain posture gives an effective stretch and stimulates neuromuscular energy. Performed carefully, it will both calm and energize.*

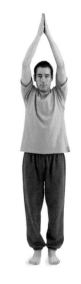

1 *Stand comfortably erect, with your feet some 3 inches apart and your hands by your sides. Turn your hands so the palms face the front. Breathing in, bring your arms slowly upward and rest your hands on the crown of your head with the palms together. Now breathe out, holding this position.*

2 *On the next in-breath slowly stretch your arms up into the air, keeping the palms together. Stretch as high as you can, holding your breath. After a few seconds bring your hands back onto your head.*

3 *Repeat the stretch movement, say five times, coordinating your breath with the slow, controlled movements. Finally, on an out-breath, bring your arms down until your hands are at chest level, palms remaining together. In this prayer position, called namaste, close your eyes, breathe quietly, and repeat to yourself several times the word "peace." On an out-breath, bring your arms slowly down to the sides.*

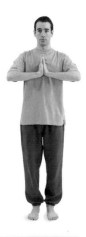

4 *Stretch up, slowly and carefully, while quietly visualizing a mountain peak, some half a dozen times.*

WORKING ON FLEXIBILITY

Now work on enhancing the flexibility of your whole body in the same standing position.

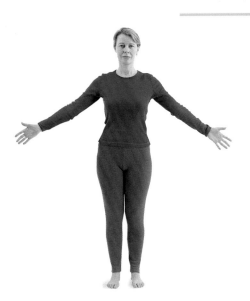

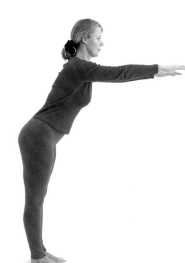

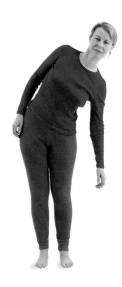

1 *Stand comfortably erect with your arms hanging by your sides. Breathe out deeply. With a slow in-breath, raise your arms out from your sides, stretching upward as your breath stops.*

2 *Breathe out, stretching your arms and trunk forward, trying not to bend your back.*

3 *On the in-breath, swing your arms upward again and bend backward, allowing your knees to bend to maintain the balance.*

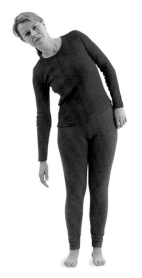

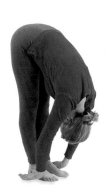

4 *Straighten up, breathing out. Breathe in, holding the upright position. On the next out-breath bend from the hips to the right.*

5 *Keeping the breathing rhythm, repeat step 4 to the left, then stretch upward once more.*

6 *Breathe out, slowly bringing your arms down to your sides. Now, with a slightly faster breathing rhythm, let the body above the hips go slack and swing from side to side. Stand with your eyes closed for a few moments without moving. You will feel calm but refreshed.*

All-over Stretches

··

*Stretching releases tension in the muscles and improves their tone by
stimulating local blood flow and restoring their biochemical balance.
A sequence of exercises aimed at stretching the body's major muscle groups
will also improve mental alertness. Combined with effective breathing,
stretching will stimulate the flow of energy through the whole body.*

Stretching as a preparation for the asanas should not be too vigorous. The aim is not to work out but to prepare the body for stronger exercise. At this stage the body is still easing into exercising, and loading tension onto the muscles could be damaging. Stretching can be very gentle and it can be carried out in any position – sitting or even lying on the floor (see pages 160–61), as well as standing. The postures shown on these two pages are an unusual combination of comfortable stretching and energized breathing. This makes them particularly suitable for preparing the mind and the body for a balanced session of working on asanas. The standing exercise also presents a way of enhancing the breathing while easing the spine and freeing the back muscles.

There are times when even a normally energetic person feels unusually stiff, mentally as well as physically. When this happens, instead of forcing the body it is sensible and practical to begin exercising while sitting in a chair. This often arouses a strong flow of energy, which can be the impetus to stand up and work with the whole body.

Bear in mind that whatever form of movement you attempt, the mind and body need to be eased into it for the result to be successful. Simple stretching combined with energized breathing can be practiced sitting on the side of the bed or in a bedside chair or standing in front of an open window first thing in the morning. This is also an excellent preparation for the vigorous activity the body might perform during the day.

SITTING STRETCHES

1 *Sit comfortably erect, breathe out slowly through the nose then, breathing in, swing your arms into the air, stretching upward. Hold the stretch for a few seconds.*

2 *Breathing out quite sharply through the nose, swing forward, letting your arms collapse downward until your fingers touch the ground. Swing your head from side to side to release tension in the neck. Hold this position for several seconds.*

3 *Repeat steps 1 and 2 up to 12 times. Afterward, sit quietly for a minute or two, eyes closed, your hands together in your lap.*

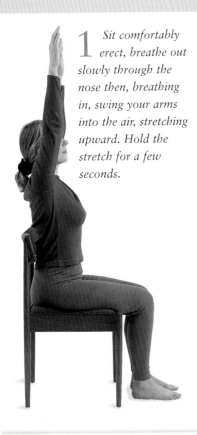
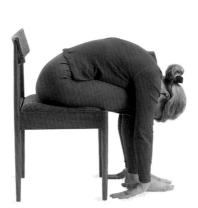
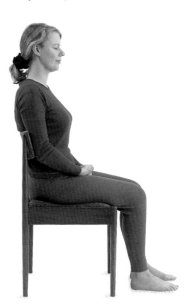

STANDING STRETCHES

1 Stand erect with the feet about 12 inches apart. Breathe out and then, breathing in slowly, swing your arms up into the air over your head, thrusting your hips forward. Hold this position for a few seconds.

3 On an in-breath, straighten up, place your hands behind your back, and, continuing to breathe in, let your trunk and shoulders swing back as far as possible without straining. Hold for about a minute, breathing through the nose. Drop your arms. Repeat steps 1–3 two or three times.

2 While bending forward and swinging the arms downward, breathe out through the mouth, making a long "Ha" sound. Bend only as far as comfortably possible and let your arms hang. Do not strain in any way. Now breathe slowly and gently through the nose. Hold the position for a minute.

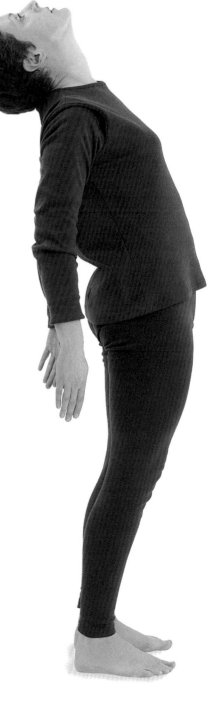

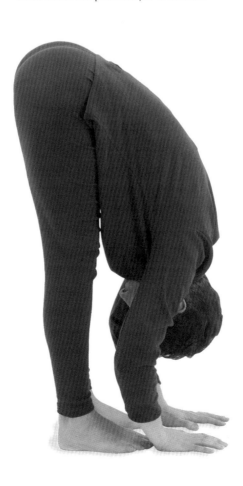

Stretching Head, Neck, and Shoulders

These days, almost everyone spends a great deal of every day sitting. This is especially true of Western cultures, where all too often people sit in a hunched-up position not only when resting and watching television but also while driving or riding on a bus or a train, and at work. In the past most people, including children, worked in the open air, on the land, doing things that utilized the whole body. Today, most people's jobs involve long periods of sitting and performing repetitive tasks. Clearly, this major change in lifestyle is putting great stresses on the body, and a wide range of illnesses may result.

Prevention is the best solution to illnesses resulting from misuse of the body, and since people spend so much time seated, making an effort never to sit in an unnatural position is good preventive medicine. The body is designed to sit with the shoulders back and the neck and head upright and balanced. Sitting hunched up – with the shoulders up and the neck and head leaning forward – tenses the neck and shoulder muscles. At first, this just causes stiffness, but in time the neck bones become affected and pain may develop.

People will often take a brief stretch to relieve discomfort after sitting immobile. But stretching while half-lying on a sofa or getting up out of an office chair, with the back inclined at an unnatural angle, the neck bent forward, and the limbs askew is more likely to cause damage than bring relief. Stretching imposes stresses on bones, joints, tendons, and muscles. To relieve tension in the head, neck, and shoulders – as in any other part of the body – it is important to begin by sitting or standing erect, so that the body is balanced and the bones are aligned correctly. The exercises illustrated below and on pages 64–67 and 70–71 show how to stretch most effectively to relieve tension in the upper body.

SHOULDER-SHRUGGING

If your shoulders feel tense, just shrugging them a few times will free the muscles and relieve some of the tension. This exercise can be done while you are standing or sitting. Performed regularly, it will can relieve chronic stiffness in either or both of the shoulders.

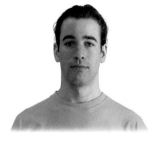

1 *Stand or sit with your back erect but not stiff and your head well balanced, eyes facing forward, arms by your sides.*

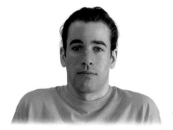

2 *While breathing in, lift both shoulders up toward your ears. Breathe out, letting your shoulders fall quickly back to their natural position. Repeat step 2 three or four times.*

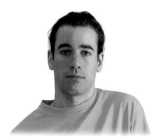

3 *Repeat step 2 lifting only the left shoulder, then only the right shoulder, breathing in each time you lift a shoulder and out as you drop it. Repeat step 3 three or four times.*

EXERCISING THE NECK

These exercises are an effective restorative for whenever the neck feels stiff.

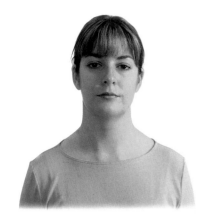

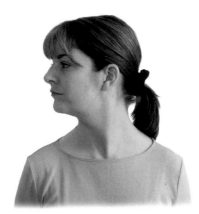

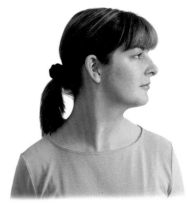

1 Sit in a chair with your lower back pressing against the chair back and your head up and facing forward. Your arms should hang loosely by your sides so that your shoulders fall into a natural position.

2 Breathe in, then breathe out, turning your head slowly to the right; stop turning as the last of the air is expelled. Hold the position and breathe in, then breathe out slowly again and try to turn your head further to the right. Breathe in slowly.

3 Breathing out, turn your head slowly to the left, and stop turning as the last of the air is expelled. You should be facing forward when you need to breathe in. Take several slow, deep breaths to help relax the muscles.

4 Repeat step 2, turning your head to the left. Then repeat step 3 until you face forward again. Take several slow, deep breaths.

5 On an out-breath, let your chin fall to rest on your chest. Breathe in and out rhythmically, lowering your head a little more with each out-breath.

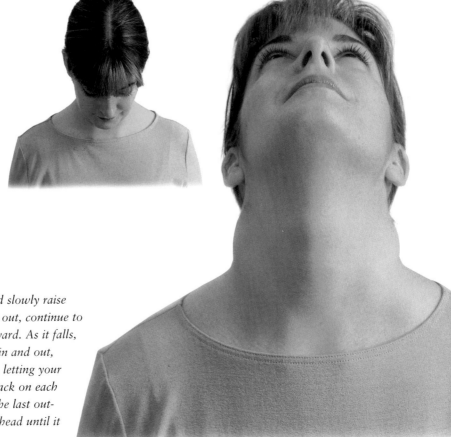

6 Take an in-breath and slowly raise your head. Breathing out, continue to raise it until it falls backward. As it falls, clench your jaw. Breathe in and out, keeping the jaw clenched, letting your head fall a little further back on each out-breath. As you take the last out-breath, slowly raise your head until it faces forward again.

Stretching Arms, Trunk, and Legs

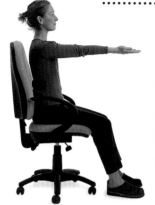

Stretching may prevent the onset of repetitive strain injury.

Although there are asanas to exercise virtually every muscle in the body, a short yoga session will usually focus on a certain group of asanas aimed at increasing the flexibility of the back, for example, or working on shoulder stands, so that some parts of the body may be temporarily neglected. Devoting preliminary warm-up time to exercising the arms and abdomen and the hips and legs achieves a balanced approach, which is the major aim of yoga practice.

Anyone who has been largely immobile for most of the day will particularly benefit from and enjoy simple exercises to stretch and rotate the legs and arms. Arm stretches are especially beneficial for anyone who works at a keyboard, since they help prevent RSI (repetitive strain injury). People with this condition experience pain when they use their hands. It results from repetitive use of a keyboard over a long period, which damages the nerves and muscles of the arms and hands. The exercises illustrated here will all stretch and tone the muscles of the chest, the abdomen, and the limbs, hands, and feet, improving their circulation and muscle tone.

As long as they are carried out with the correct breathing, the mountain posture illustrated on page 64, the flexibility exercises on page 66, and the hip wiggle illustrated opposite will also help to ease stiffness in the lower back. All these exercises are suitable for anyone who suffers from recurrent lower back pain, although it is wise to do them very gently, relaxing immediately if any pain is experienced. Done regularly as part of yoga practice they will stretch and gradually realign the lumbar vertebrae (the bones of the lower part of the spine), and so ease chronic back pain, and they will prevent serious conditions such as a slipped disk from ever developing.

ARM STRETCH

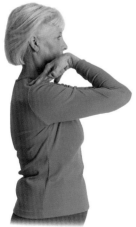

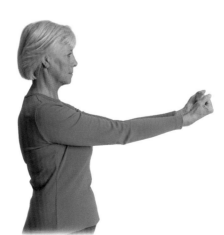

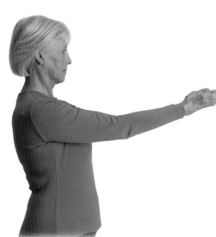

1 *Stand, or sit in a chair, with the trunk comfortably erect. Stretch your arms out in front of you with the palms facing upward, then place your fingertips on your shoulders. On an out-breath sharply stretch your arms and hands out to the front.*

2 *With your arms still outstretched, fold your fingers in to make fists, then snap your fingers out.*

3 *Repeat steps 1 and 2 about ten times. Finish by letting your hands go limp and shaking them in the air for a few minutes.*

HIP WIGGLE

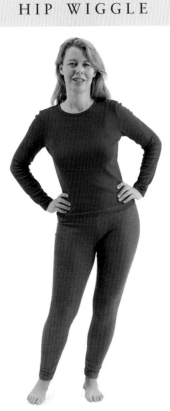

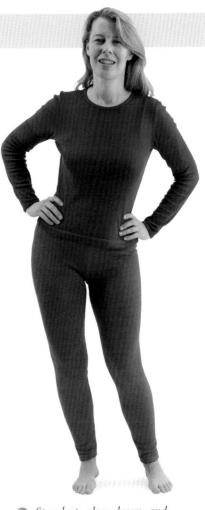

1 Stand with your feet a shoulder width apart and rest your hands on your hips. Bend your knees slightly.

CAUTION
....

If you suffer from lower back pain or a slipped disk do not attempt this exercise.

2 Move your right hip slowly to the right, then back, then left, then forward several times until you begin to gyrate to a rhythm. Repeat, but this time start by moving your left hip to the left.

3 Speed up, slow down, and have fun wiggling and gyrating (you can do this exercise to music). Do not worry about breathing, just follow a rhythm and your breathing will adjust to your movements.

FLEXIBLE FEET

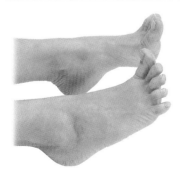

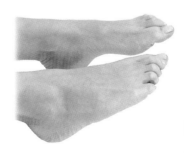

3 Bend your right leg and rest it on your left thigh. Take your right foot in your left hand and rotate it several times in each direction. Repeat the exercise with your left leg and rotate your left foot.

1 Sit on the floor with your trunk erect and your legs stretched out in front of you, feet slightly apart. Support yourself on your hands if you feel you need to. Try to separate your toes, moving each one independently of the others.

2 With your legs still out in front of you, stretch the feet forward, keeping the heels on the ground, then release and try again, two or three times.

Relaxation

....

Yoga sessions should always be punctuated by moments of stillness.
As well as a pause for controlled breathing at the beginning of a session,
body and mind need to rest between asanas – the body to recover from
exertion and the mind to clear itself, ready for the next mental task.
At the end of a session there should be a prolonged period of relaxation.

Many people find it difficult to relax, mainly because relaxation is not a skill that is widely taught at home or at school. A great deal of what is described as relaxation is in fact just flopping, the body and limbs askew, with no regard to posture. To relax, it is necessary for the body to be in a natural position – lying, sitting, even standing – so that breathing remains effective, enabling the blood circulation and the neuroelectrical system to function properly. True relaxation is described by people who practice yoga as a state of observation without intervention: someone who is really relaxing is aware of everything that is happening in the immediate surroundings but remains still, not responding to it.

At first it can be hard to let the mind go free without instantly changing the points to send it along the track that leads through the maze of daily preoccupations. Through the breathing, meditation, and visualization techniques explained in Chapters 8 and 9 people gradually learn to control the mind and prevent this from happening. The simplest technique for a beginner to use, however, is just to concentrate on relaxing each part of the body in turn, beginning with the feet and progressing up the body.

CORPSE

1 *Sit on the floor with your knees bent and your feet flat on the floor. Drop backward, resting your upper body on the elbows, forearms, and the palms of the hands.*

2 *Moving your hands and forearms forward, drop gently down onto the floor, pressing your back flat against the floor. Now slide your feet forward and press the backs of your knees against the floor. Move your legs and arms out to the sides a little and turn them outward.*

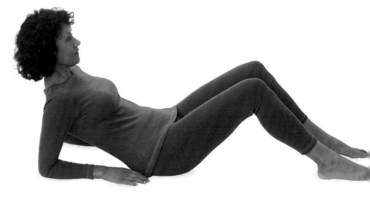

3 *Gently shut your eyes. Keep them closed as your breathing goes into a regular, shallow pattern. Beginning with the toes, relax each body part in turn. If any area seems tense, gently contract the muscles around it and let them relax again. Before your thoughts reach your head, your mind will have drifted into a pleasantly lethargic state.*

4 *When you feel you have relaxed enough, stand up slowly. At first you may find you have relaxed for 5 minutes or less, but as you become used to it the period of relaxation will lengthen to 15 minutes or more. Try to prolong the feeling of relaxation as you move to the next phase of the day.*

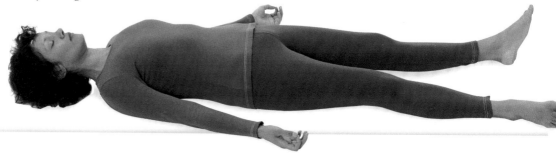

AREAS OF TENSION

Lift your head slightly and shake it to free the neck muscles, then let it fall gently back onto the mat.

Close your eyes and relax the muscles surrounding them.

Be aware of any tension in your mouth, but do not relax it so much that it falls open.

Briefly press your shoulders down toward the mat, then release.

Your rate of breathing should fall to about six breaths a minute.

Lift up your arms and briefly shake them, then let them flop back onto the mat.

The lower part of the back of your head should touch the mat. If your chin is pressed in or if your throat feels stretched, reposition your head so that it forms a straight line with your body.

If there is a gap between your lower back and the floor, bend your knees and bring your feet back until your heels touch your thighs, then gently slide your feet forward again while pressing your lower back into the mat.

Tense the abdominal muscles, then release them. As you breathe in, the abdomen should rise gently and fall again on the out-breath.

Your hands should be relaxed, palms upward, thumb and forefinger allowed to touch.

Moving your feet 12–15 inches apart relaxes your leg muscles.

Allowing your feet to fall outward enables your ankles to relax.

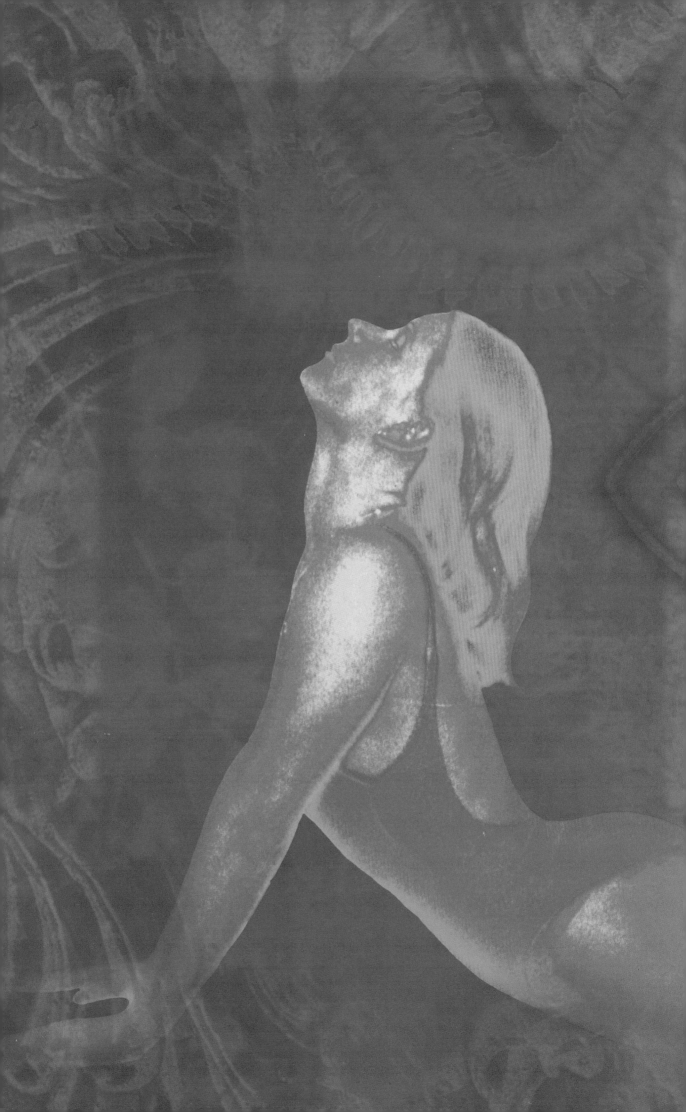

Part Six
The Positions

Beginning...

....

To a beginner, some of the yoga postures illustrated in this chapter look impossible, but although it can take years, they can be achieved. Learning them may cause a few initial aches and pains, but in time they make the body more mobile and flexible.

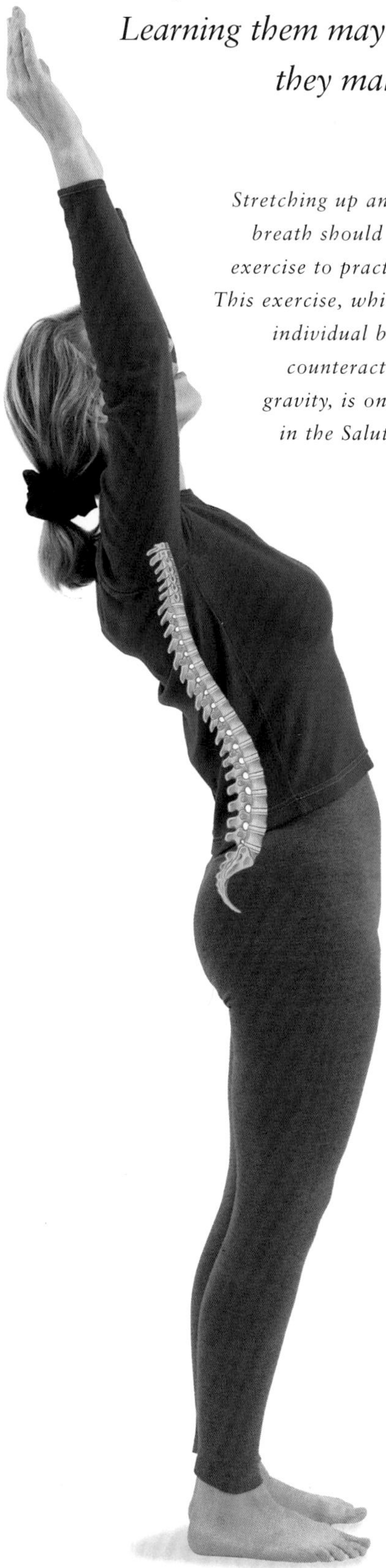

Stretching up and back on an in-breath should be a preliminary exercise to practicing the asanas. This exercise, which stretches each individual bone of the spine, counteracting the effects of gravity, is one of the postures in the Salute to the Sun (see page 99).

Starting with the circulatory system, which is energized by moving and stretching, all the body's systems are stimulated by practicing the yoga asanas. When they are accompanied by the correct breathing, and followed by relaxation, the asanas have this effect because they ease tension and improve posture. They also remove obstacles to the flow of energy and electromagnetism around the body.

It is important to always work at the body's own pace, and to treat it gently and with love. Many factors affect its functioning: cold, heat, dryness, humidity, current thoughts, and long-standing worries, and it needs to be eased into the postures.

Students who practice regularly always progress, but the speed of change can vary enormously. Improvement in one area may take days and in another it may be months or even years. Only one thing is certain: the first or last past the post always finds another post just visible ahead, because each asana leads on to progressively more difficult variations. So it is important to aim at steady progress and not to be too encouraged by signs of quick advancement or discouraged by no apparent progress.

The degree of flexibility of the spine affects the mobility of the rest of the body to a great degree, so it is essential not only to exercise the spine regularly but to work on increasing its arc of movement. The way to do this without damaging the spine is through gentle exercises that bend and stretch it backward – as shown on the left – then forward, and to either side, as shown opposite. Stretching a stiff back can be hard work, but breathing in the correct way helps stretch it a little more each time. Careful and controlled twisting, shown opposite, is also an effective way of making the spine more supple.

The bends and twists illustrated on pages 78–83 will restore flexibility to an immobile spine and help to maintain it if they are made part of regular practice. The asanas on pages 84–95 go further, increasing the mobility of the spine as a whole by exercising and strengthening the muscles that control it. They also strengthen the muscles in other parts of the body.

MOBILITY AND FLEXIBILITY

The design of the spine has been perfected through evolution for the benefit of its owner. It has been said that the spine we have today is the one that evolved millions of years ago for ancestors of modern humans who walked on all fours, and that spinal problems such as back pain and slipped disks are the inevitable consequence of humans having taken to walking upright. This is not so. As the body evolved, the spine evolved with it, adapting to human changes in mobility. The spine's S-shape is an evolved design – its curves are not kinks that need to be straightened out. Habitual slumping and lack of exercise stiffen the spine. Through yoga exercises, which stretch it in four different directions, its natural flexibility will be restored in time.

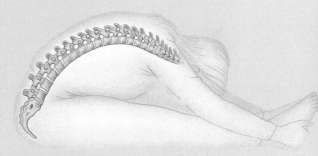

A forward bend needs to follow every exercise that bends the spine backward. This posterior stretch (see page 78) bends the spinal column forward without compressing the bones of the neck or stretching them out of alignment.

The bow posture (see page 92) stretches the front of the spinal column, separating the individual vertebrae (bones of the spine), producing an accentuated curve.

Sideways bends (see page 84) can be practiced on the left and the right to increase the sideways flexibility of the spine.

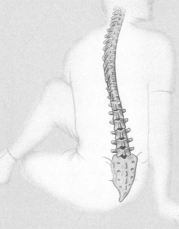

The spinal twist (see pages 80-81) stretches and lengthens every muscle and ligament of the spine and separates the vertebrae (spinal bones).

Stretching the Spine

···

The spine is not rigid. The vertebrae – the bones, some fused, others connected by ligaments, that make up the spine – work together to give the body great flexibility of movement. Slipped disks and other problems occur because the spine is not used in the way it should be. Perhaps as much as 80 percent of lower back pain is due to poor posture, and so is preventable.

If the back is exercised properly and regularly, the spine is able to do its job without the ever-present risk of damage. The ease with which people "put the back out" serves as proof of the back's need to be exercised regularly. A person who never exercises might be sitting at a desk, turn around sharply for some reason, sense an internal click, and be unable to get up. Anyone who has been exercising regularly to keep the spine flexible will never experience that problem. The same is true of other back complaints – slipped disks are the culminating disaster in a series of spinal injuries which began, most often, with bad posture that was never corrected. The stretches illustrated on the next few pages are the first steps in encouraging the spine's natural flexibility to reassert itself.

POSTERIOR STRETCH

This asana is designed to counter the compressing action of gravity on the spine. Do not try to force the spine to stretch further than it can easily go. Just follow the sequence of movements and concentrate on the breathing. With practice any stiffness will ease and your back will begin to bend more easily.

1 *Sit on the floor with your legs in front of you. Your feet should be a hand's breadth apart and pointing upward. Sit with your spine and head erect and your hands resting on the floor at your sides. Breathe slowly out, then inhale while lifting your arms right above your head and raising your trunk, stretching all the muscles of the back. Keep the backs of your legs on the floor.*

2 *Breathing out, and with your back still lifted and your arms extended upward, stretch forward slowly. Keep the backs of your legs on the floor. Concentrate your thoughts on stretching forward.*

3 *As the out-breath ends, lower your arms to grasp your legs as far down as you can reach – the calves, the ankles, the toes. Drop your head and relax for at least half a minute, breathing gently while continuing to stretch.*

COBRA

*This bend, which imitates the rearing movement
of a cobra, stretches the front of the body and
counterbalances the posterior stretch.*

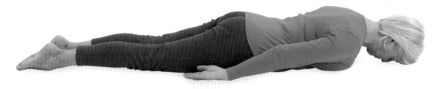

1 Lie face down, with your forehead
resting on the mat and your arms
by your sides, palms upward. Breathe
out slowly.

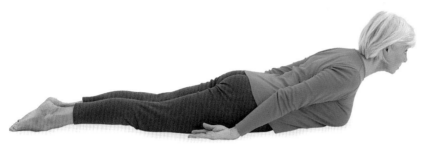

2 Breathe in, lifting first your head,
then your neck, shoulders, and
chest from the mat.

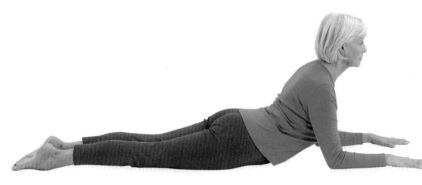

3 As soon as you feel you have lifted
your head as far as you can, or if
your back is weak or has been injured,
move your arms forward so that you
rest on your forearms, palms down.

4 On an in-breath, continue to lift the upper body while
keeping your hips and legs on the floor. When you feel
able, straighten your arms and rest your weight on the
palms of your hands. Close your eyes and breathe slowly
for at least half a minute. Then, breathing out, slowly
lower the upper body and move your arms back to your
sides, until you are lying as you were in step 1. Relax.

5 Repeat steps 1–4 at each daily practice. Concentrate
on your breathing and on stretching a little further
back each time. As your spine becomes more flexible
you will find you move your hands gradually closer
to your body.

Performing the Spinal Twist

The spinal twist stretches and lengthens every muscle and ligament of the spine, increasing the flow of blood to that area and toning the muscles, making it more supple. The full twist is difficult, and beginners are traditionally taught it in stages, progressing from the simple twist and the half twist.

What makes the spinal twist special is that instead of bending and stretching the spine it turns each vertebra on its axis, twisting the spine along its entire length, from the sacrum (the lower vertebrae) to the skull. It is also unusual in that it starts from a sitting position. The pelvis does not rotate and the shoulders do most of the work: as they turn, the spine follows. Nothing in yoga is entirely physical and the success of this posture depends on correct breathing – the twist takes place during exhalation. The mind must concentrate on relaxing the muscles of the spine to achieve as complete a twist as possible.

The best thing about this asana is that, performed correctly, with attention to breathing, it tones up the nerves of the spinal cord and stimulates the whole body. It helps you to become more supple and creates an immediate feeling of well-being. People who suffer from back pain can benefit from doing these exercises, but they must ease into them very slowly and stop immediately if the exercise causes any pain.

SIMPLE SPINAL TWIST

This simple variant of the spinal twist helps mobilize a stiff spine. If you find this asana difficult, concentrate on breathing correctly while working on turning your shoulders a little further than you think they will go. After you finish, lie and relax for a few minutes.

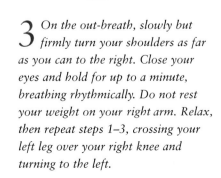

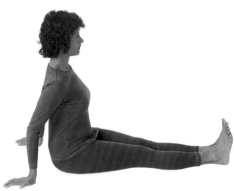

1 *Sit with your legs out in front of you and your feet together, toes pointing upward. Do not slump backward; instead, lift your trunk and sit upright, but without creating strain in the muscles of the back.*

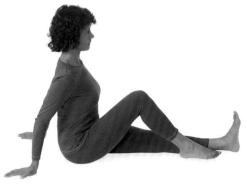

2 *Touch your spine with your right hand, then drop your hand onto the mat level with it. Cross your right leg over your left leg at the knee joint, and stretch your left arm outward, pressing your elbow against the right side of your right knee. Breathe in.*

3 *On the out-breath, slowly but firmly turn your shoulders as far as you can to the right. Close your eyes and hold for up to a minute, breathing rhythmically. Do not rest your weight on your right arm. Relax, then repeat steps 1–3, crossing your left leg over your right knee and turning to the left.*

HALF TWIST

When you are performing the simple spinal twist without difficulty and you feel your spine is now more flexible, try the half twist, in which both legs are bent. Your movements should be slow at first, until you are confident you have the details right, but at the point when you begin to hold the position, clear your mind and keep it still by visualizing something peaceful.

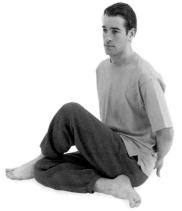

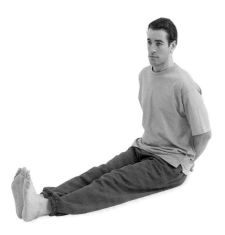

3 Now place your right arm diagonally across your chest. The elbow should press against your bent left knee. Breathe in. On the out-breath, slowly but firmly turn your shoulders to the left. Keeping the right knee touching the floor, and without lifting either hip, turn your shoulders as far as they will go.

1 Sit upright with your legs out in front of you, touch your spine with your left hand, then drop your hand onto the mat level with it, palm downward, a few inches away from your lower back. Do not rest your weight on this hand.

2 Bend your right leg keeping the knee touching the floor and pressing the heel into your groin. Cross your left leg over your right leg at the knee joint, resting the left foot on the mat touching your right knee.

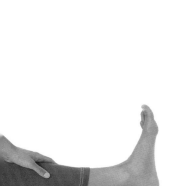

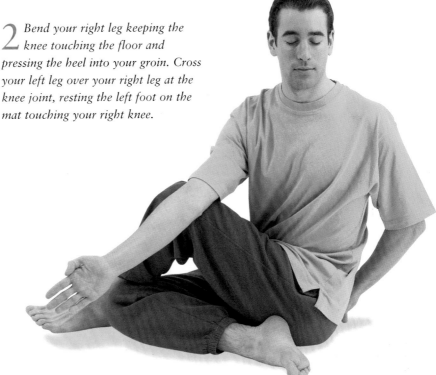

4 Close your eyes and breathe rhythmically for about two minutes, holding the position and keeping your mind still. Try to keep your spine erect through your own muscle power – do not rest your weight on your left arm. Turn your shoulders and then your arms to the front, uncross your legs, and resume the sitting position you adopted in step 1. Relax and repeat the exercise, this time bending your left leg and crossing your right leg over your left knee.

Bending the Spine

···

The spine can bend in four directions. First, it can bend forward. In yoga, however, the spine is never allowed to collapse forward, as if someone had loaded a heavy weight onto the back of the shoulders. Instead, it is stretched forward so that the whole of the trunk is lifted. This counters gravity, taking the pressure off the vertebrae – for a short time. And in yoga, a forward bend does not stretch the spine alone but the whole posterior side of the body.

To maintain balance and encourage flexibility, an exercise to bend the spine backward always follows a forward bend. It is not as easy to stretch the spine back as it is to bend it forward. Because it is something that people do very infrequently in everyday life, students often find it harder to bend backward than to bend forward. However, it is essential to work on backward bends. To remain healthy and active, all parts of the body need to be exercised regularly. Stretching the spine keeps it flexible and counters the compressing effect that gravity has on it. Everyone, no matter how young or old, can benefit from spinal exercises, for without exercise the spine will not function properly, so that after years of disuse, people lose flexibility to the extent that they find it difficult to bend in any direction.

Illustrated on the following two pages are exercises to increase the spine's flexibility still further, by increasing its natural capacity to bend sideways, as well as backward and forward.

STANDING BACKWARD BEND

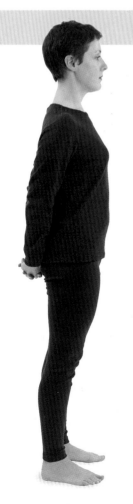

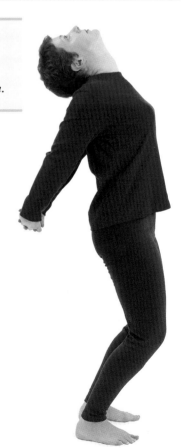

This simple backward bend contracts the back muscles and stretches the muscles of the thighs, the abdomen, the chest, and the throat. Relax the muscles of your shoulders and back before you begin.

1 *Stand erect with your feet at shoulder's width apart and your arms relaxed by your sides. Link your fingers behind your back. Now breathe in and, bending your knees slightly, swing your arms well back and let your head fall backward. Feel the stretch in your thighs, abdomen, and throat.*

2 *On the out-breath slowly draw your linked hands back toward your body, raise your head, and straighten your knees.*

3 *Repeat steps 1 and 2 three times.*

TOUCHING YOUR TOES

Performed properly, this exercise stretches the entire body and stimulates the mind, but to try to force the back to bend to its fullest extent in one jerk, unaided by correct breathing, could cause injury. In yoga, touching the toes is the last movement in this smoothly executed sequence governed by effective breathing.

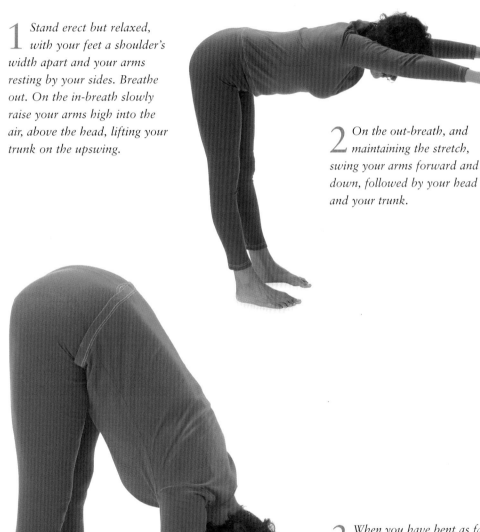

1 *Stand erect but relaxed, with your feet a shoulder's width apart and your arms resting by your sides. Breathe out. On the in-breath slowly raise your arms high into the air, above the head, lifting your trunk on the upswing.*

2 *On the out-breath, and maintaining the stretch, swing your arms forward and down, followed by your head and your trunk.*

3 *When you have bent as far forward as you can, try to touch the floor with your fingers, then hold the position for at least one minute, breathing slowly and silently. Shake your head gently to release any latent tension in your neck. Breathe in and lift your body, starting from the hips, followed by the chest, shoulders, head, and the arms and hands, as if you were slowly unrolling. Breathe out and then lower your arms to your sides.*

Sideways Movement

··

Almost everyone thinks they can bend sideways with ease, but when they try they often find to their dismay that flexibility in that direction is less than they expected. A jerky sideways bend to pick up something from a low table or a chair can result in a day or more of intense pain in the lower back for anyone with a spine that has become inflexible through disuse.

Maintaining the capacity for sideways movement is essential if the spine is to remain supple. Moreover, sideways bends are a good way of alternately stretching and compressing each side of the chest and the abdomen, increasing the blood circulation to the internal organs and enabling the chest and lungs to expand more easily. The exercises illustrated here tense and so strengthen the waist and neck, making them more flexible.

Everybody is different and some students find they can bend easily from side to side, while others can bend only about 2 inches to either side. Students who find sideways bends difficult should work on them as part of their daily yoga program, doing each exercise slowly and thoroughly. As always, good posture is essential, and breathing is the key to progress. Having bent so far, breathe gently for a while to achieve a calm and focused state of mind, and try to bend a little more before resting.

SIDEWAYS BEND

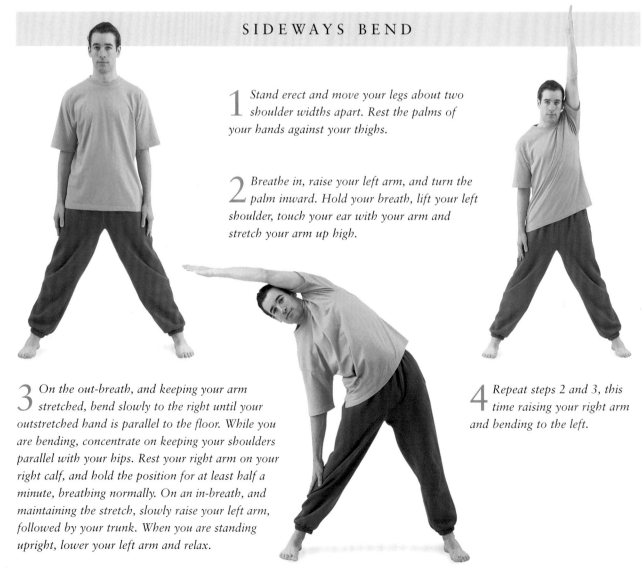

1 *Stand erect and move your legs about two shoulder widths apart. Rest the palms of your hands against your thighs.*

2 *Breathe in, raise your left arm, and turn the palm inward. Hold your breath, lift your left shoulder, touch your ear with your arm and stretch your arm up high.*

3 *On the out-breath, and keeping your arm stretched, bend slowly to the right until your outstretched hand is parallel to the floor. While you are bending, concentrate on keeping your shoulders parallel with your hips. Rest your right arm on your right calf, and hold the position for at least half a minute, breathing normally. On an in-breath, and maintaining the stretch, slowly raise your left arm, followed by your trunk. When you are standing upright, lower your left arm and relax.*

4 *Repeat steps 2 and 3, this time raising your right arm and bending to the left.*

TRIANGLE

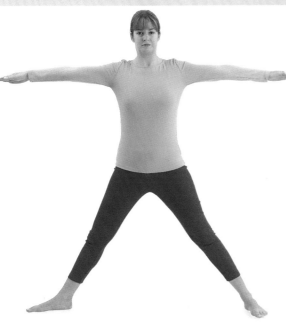

Once you can execute the sideways bend without difficulty, it is time to move on to the triangle. This asana is not easy, and beginners usually aim at creating an almost vertical line with the two outstretched arms. Accomplished yogis can bend much further to the side, so that they are almost parallel to the floor.

1 Stand erect and move your feet about two shoulder widths apart. Rotate the right foot so that it points sideways, at a right angle to the left foot; then move the toes of your left foot a little to the right. Breathe in slowly and stretch both arms out to the sides until they are parallel with the floor.

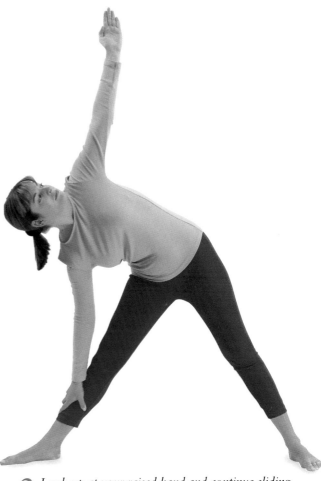

3 Look up at your raised hand and continue sliding your right hand down your calf and rest it on, or hold, your ankle. Do not twist your left shoulder forward in order to lower your hand further. Breathe gently and hold the position for as long as you can.

4 On an in-breath, turn your head to face forward, slowly lift your trunk and your right arm, and simultaneously lower your left arm until you are standing as in step 1. Breathing out, lower your arms to rest on your thighs and turn both feet to face the front. Relax.

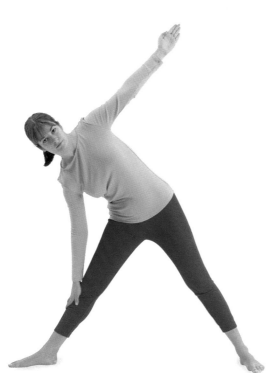

2 Breathing out, lower the right hand until it touches your thigh, then slide it down your calf. At the same time, raise your left hand high into the air and turn the palm of your hand to face the front. Keep your head in line with your trunk as you bend to the right, and keep your shoulders parallel with your hips.

5 Repeat steps 1–4, reversing the positions of the feet and this time bending to the left.

Cat and Dog

....

The asanas illustrated on the next few pages aim at improving flexibility. Some may seem advanced and difficult, but the secret is to ease the body into new postures and to aim at very gradual progress. It is futile to try to force the body to do anything difficult. Its response will be to tense up, which puts the goal of improving flexibility further into the distance.

Yoga never tries to impose its own conditions on the body, but to remove obstacles that prevent it from achieving greater flexibility for itself. To work on a part of it really means finding out what the body is able to do in that area, and satisfying its need.

This idea may seem strange to anyone who has never tried yoga, and the results may be surprising. Where the will might want the body to stick to some simple exercise, the body, in league with the unconscious, might express an urge to attempt some asana thought to be much too advanced.

Learning how to listen to the body and interpret its needs is part of learning yoga. It involves trying to release the consciousness from its tendency to try to control the body. This can be

achieved by doing something as simple as lying in the relaxation position, breathing gently and clearing the mind of everyday preoccupations, then waiting until the body's own program becomes clear.

Cats are so elastic when they stretch that they make an ideal model for a back-stretching exercise. The cat pose relieves tiredness in the back at the end of a long day. The stretch releases tension and the relaxation position is very comfortable. The pose makes the spine more flexible, restores mobility to the diaphragm, and teaches control of the abdominal muscles while breathing.

The dog pose counterbalances the forward bend of the cat pose by thrusting the body into an inverted V-shape, stretching the lower body.

CAT

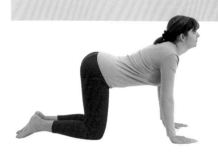

1 *Kneel with your legs a shoulder width apart. Breathing out, place your hand on the mat beneath your shoulders. Breathing in, lower your back and raise your head. Hold the position.*

Carried out every day, this simple exercise helps a rigid spine become more mobile. The breathing is important, and not only to aid relaxation and concentration. It also teaches control of the abdominal muscles. After breathing out in step 2, tuck your head between your arms and contract your stomach muscles, keeping them contracted as long as you hold your breath.

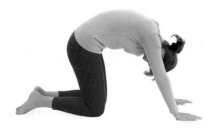

2 *Breathe out and simultaneously arch your back as high as you can while dropping your head between your arms. Hold the position and your breath for a few seconds.*

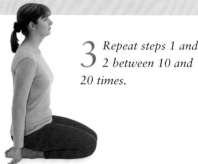

3 *Repeat steps 1 and 2 between 10 and 20 times.*

4 *Sit back on your heels while moving your arms back, resting your hands, palms up, beside your heels. Lower your head until your forehead touches the mat. Relax, breathing gently, for two or three minutes, before getting up slowly.*

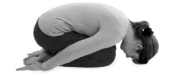

DOG

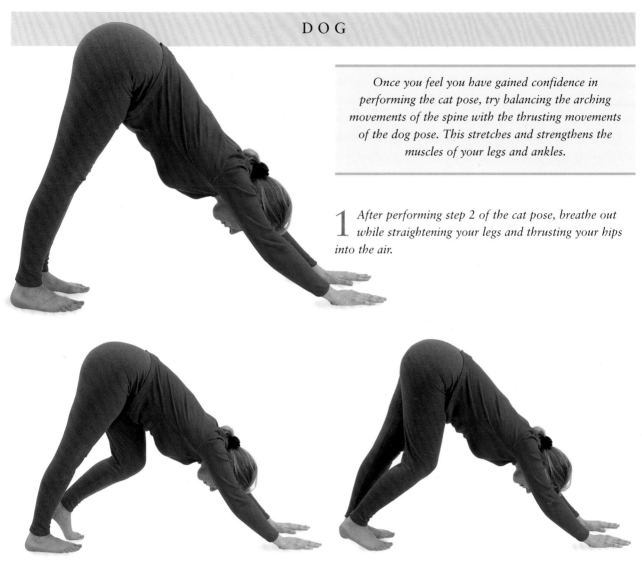

Once you feel you have gained confidence in performing the cat pose, try balancing the arching movements of the spine with the thrusting movements of the dog pose. This stretches and strengthens the muscles of your legs and ankles.

1 *After performing step 2 of the cat pose, breathe out while straightening your legs and thrusting your hips into the air.*

2 *Raise your left heel and bend the knee while pressing your right heel against the mat.*

3 *Then raise your right heel and bend the knee while pressing your left heel against the mat. Sink into the rest position and relax.*

MAKING PROGRESS

After you have been practicing the cat pose exercise for some weeks or even months and you feel that your spine is becoming more supple, you should work harder on the exercise to achieve maximum spinal movement. When you feel you have gained mobility in your spine, you will find that the controlled movements strengthen the muscles of your back and trunk.

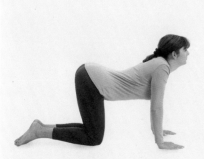

Assume the starting position for the cat on all fours (see step 1), breathe in and, while dropping your back, open your chest and swing your head and neck up.

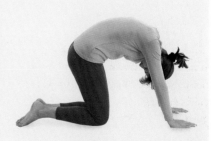

Without pausing or holding your breath, arch your back as high as it will go, while lowering your head well between your shoulders.

Bridge and Boat

··

Both the bridge and the boat stretch and exercise the muscle groups of the thighs, the buttocks, and the abdomen. They also train the sense of balance, which is often quite poor in students who have not taken part in any physical activities for some time.

Since they test and exercise such key functions, these two exercises are often difficult for students to execute when they first begin to practice yoga. They may find themselves unable to raise their trunk or legs, or find it impossible to hold a particular position for more than a second without collapsing. As with all yoga postures, breathing and effective relaxation are the secret. If the muscles are tensed and painfully strained they cannot function.

After a posture fails, it can be helpful to lie quietly for a few minutes, breathing gently and bringing the mind under control, before trying again – this time visualizing success. There is no particular virtue in being able to perform an asana with ease the first time you try. Progress may seem to be painfully slow at the beginning, but regular stretching and use makes the muscles more malleable and this helps to bring them under control.

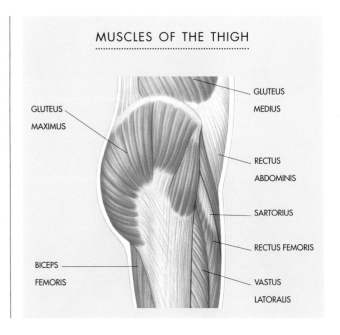

MUSCLES OF THE THIGH
··························

GLUTEUS MAXIMUS
GLUTEUS MEDIUS
RECTUS ABDOMINIS
SARTORIUS
RECTUS FEMORIS
BICEPS FEMORIS
VASTUS LATORALIS

BRIDGE

Try this exercise only when you are sure you have gained some mobility in your back. It can seem very difficult at first, but carried out effectively over time it will greatly improve the suppleness of your back.

The bridge is a good remedial exercise for anyone with lower back problems, but do not attempt it if you have pain or other problems in the upper part of the back, or in the neck or throat.

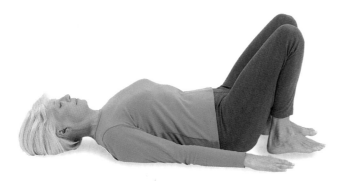

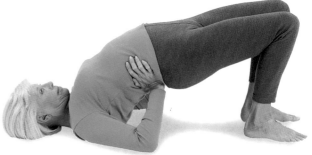

1 *Lie on your back with your head in line with your body and your arms by your sides, palms down. Bend your knees and draw your heels as close as you can to your buttocks, keeping your heels on the floor. Breathe out.*

2 *On the in-breath raise your back. Bend your elbows and slide your palms beneath the small of your back. Keeping your heels on the floor, lift your chest, and hold your breath briefly. As you breathe out, lower your hands and your back.*

BOAT

*This pose exercises and strengthens the muscles
of the thighs and the abdomen, and it makes an
excellent counterbalance to the bridge. It also
improves balance. It is important to be relaxed before
you begin and to concentrate on maintaining rhythmic
breathing throughout.*

1 *Lie on your back with your legs and feet together and
your arms by your sides, palms down. Breathe out.*

2 *Breathing in, swing your legs
up, then breathe normally for
a few moments.*

3 *Breathing in, lift your head, shoulders, and trunk off
the mat, so that you are balancing on the base of your
spine. Your outstretched fingers should rest on either side
of your legs. Hold the position and your breath for a few
seconds, then as you breathe out, lower your trunk and
head and then your legs onto the mat. Rest, breathing
gently for a few seconds.*

4 *Repeat step 3 three times, remembering to lift as you
breathe out. Try to keep your mind relaxed, so that
you hold the position for a second or two longer each time,
but breathe out and rest if your abdominal muscles begin
to shudder.*

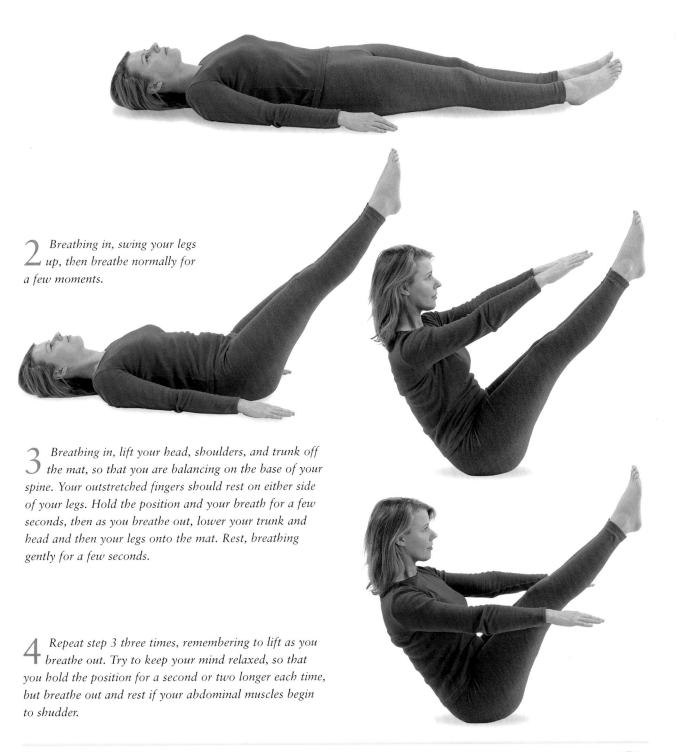

Learning Effective Muscle Control

Because the spine runs the length of the trunk and abdomen, most movements designed to exercise it stimulate and, therefore, benefit the internal organs.

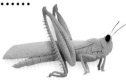

The shape of the locust is what gives the asana on the facing page its name.

Postures such as the fish stimulate the kidneys, intestines, spleen, liver, and lungs, and the ovaries and uterus in women. This increases the flow of blood in those areas as well as the action of the stomach and intestines, speeding the digestive process. Postures such as the locust stretch the solar plexus – the nerve center located in the region of the stomach – whose function is often distorted by repeated anxiety. Deep breathing combined with stretching increase the blood flow to that area and soothe the nerves, inducing a sense of calm. The bow (see page 92), which arches the neck, also brings about relaxation. Even just attempting many of these postures releases immediate feelings of well-being.

However, the primary purpose of practicing the two exercises here is to maximize the mobility of the spine and to learn effective muscle control. The fish exercises the underused muscles of the neck. The locust calls for control over a group of muscles called the *Lattismus dorsii* in the small of the back. These muscles are exercised so rarely that learning to use and strengthen them may take a few weeks.

FISH

Tradition has it that in ancient times this posture was named the fish (the translation of its Sanskrit name) because it allows the body to float in water while enabling it to breathe. It is more commonly practiced as a counterposture to the plow and the half-candle (see pages 94–96).

1 *Lie on the floor with your legs and feet together and your arms by your sides, palms down. On an in-breath, raise your trunk and simultaneously move your arms back and bend the elbows so they support your shoulders. Hollow your back as deeply as you can, at the same time letting your head fall back.*

2 *Holding your breath, move your elbows slowly outward until the crown of your head rests on the floor. Keep your buttocks on the floor.*

3 *Raise your arms, bringing the palms of your hands together on your chest in the gesture of prayer called namaste. Concentrate on breathing slowly and deeply, and hold the position for about 30 seconds. On an out-breath, relax your back, align your head and neck with your body, and rest.*

CAUTION

If this asana makes you feel giddy or nauseous, stop immediately and do not attempt it again without consulting a physician.

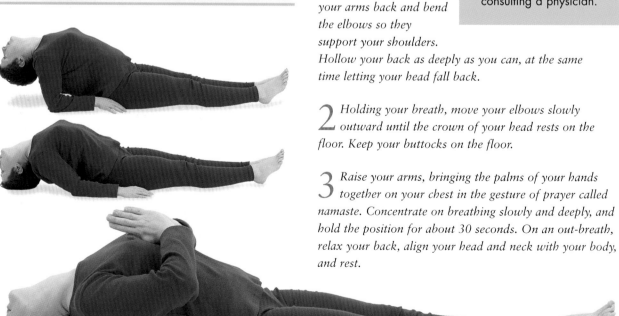

LOCUST

To perform this asana successfully, concentrate on every muscle being exercised. Keep the raised leg straight and do not tense the calves or point the toes vigorously; your feet should be relaxed and at an angle to your calves. Try to remain relaxed, even if you can sustain the posture only for a second or two.

1 *Lie face down, with your forehead resting on the mat, your legs out behind you, the soles of your feet facing upward, and your arms by your sides, palms downward. Stretch your neck, pushing your chin as far forward as possible, so that it rests on the mat. Breathe out slowly.*

2 *Breathe in, and leaning slightly on your left arm, contract the muscles in the small of your back and lift your left leg from the mat. It is important to keep your pelvis on the mat and not to twist it and to keep your left arm from shoulder to fingertips firmly on the mat. Keep your left leg straight as you lift it. Hold the position for a few seconds, then lower your leg as you breathe out. Repeat this step with the right leg.*

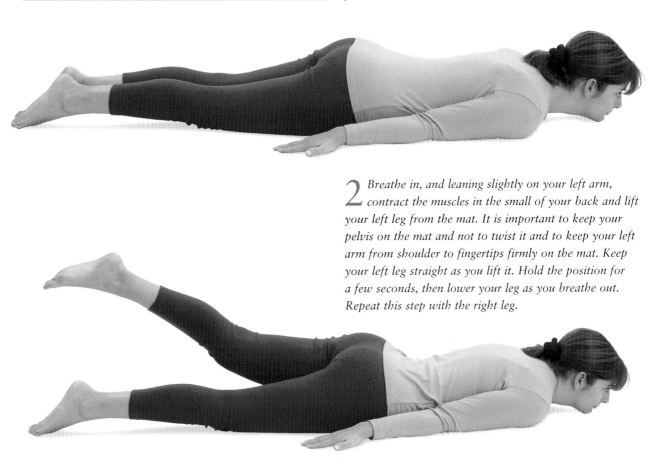

3 *Only when you can perform steps 1and 2, the half locust, without straining should you go onto the full locust. Repeat step 1 in all details, but this time clench your fists. Breathing in, contract the muscles in the small of your back and raise both legs simultaneously. Do not bend your knees, stiffen your calves, or point your toes. Keep your chin on the mat and try to keep your shoulders touching the mat while you hold the position. Breathing out, lower your legs and unclench your fists. Rest and then repeat.*

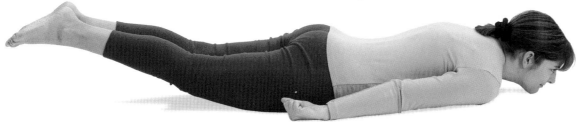

Maintaining Balance

....

Some people find these asanas fairly easy to master, but others might find that they cannot even achieve the first steps. The first stage in tackling the difficulty successfully is to understand that adopting a positive approach to a problem is as much a part of yoga as a perfectly executed asana.

Muscle groups that are unused to being stretched, such as the abdominal muscles, must be treated gently. They will quickly reach the limit of their extension, but may be induced to stretch a little more after being held in tension for a few seconds. Jerking movements and straining will only damage them.

Spend several days just on the preliminary steps of a difficult pose or in breaking down an exercise such as the pose of tranquility into two or three stages. When you feel confident about executing these steps, apply yourself to the whole asana. The goal is to progress from step to step in smooth movements, breathing correctly, instead of trying to force the pace.

This posture is named after the shape of a drawn bow.

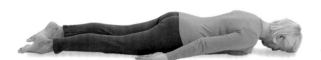

BOW

The breathing technique adopted in this pose is different from usual. Instead of breathing in when you lift your trunk, you breathe out. This causes you to pull at the moment when your muscles are relaxing, which helps them to stretch to their maximum extent.

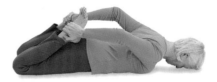

1 *Lie face down on the mat with your legs and feet together and your arms by your sides, palms up. Breathe out.*

2 *Breathing in, bend your knees and grasp your ankles with your hands, then bend your legs until your heels touch your buttocks.*

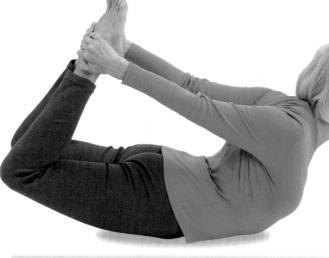

3 *Breathe out, breathe in, then take a long out-breath, at the same time lifting your head, shoulders, and chest, and pulling your ankles toward your head so that you lift your calves and thighs from the floor. Hold the out-breath for a few seconds, resting on your waist, then slowly lower your chest, shoulders, and head to rest on the mat, and breathe in.*

4 *Repeat step 3 three times, remembering to lift your body as you breathe out. Concentrate on keeping your mind relaxed so that you do not generate a sense of strain.*

POSE OF TRANQUILITY

1 Lie on the floor with your legs and feet together, toes pointing up, and your arms by your sides, palms down. Move your head forward so that your chin points toward your chest. If your lower back is not touching the floor, bend your legs, press your back into the floor, and lower your legs again. Relax and breathe out deeply.

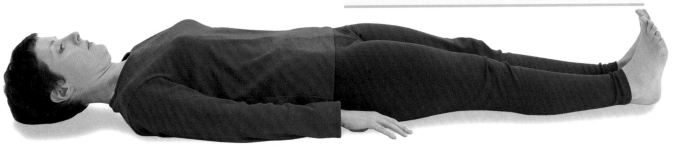

In this exercise it is important to keep both legs straight and raise them together, slowly, without making any scissor movement. Use your stomach muscles to raise your legs – do not tense the muscles of the calves or thighs, do not point your feet, and do not use your arm muscles to help raise your legs. Throughout this posture you should breathe normally and calmly.

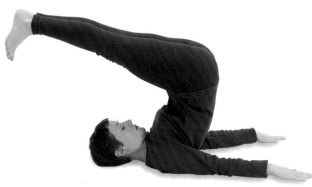

2 On the in-breath swing your legs into the air. You can then use your outstretched arms and hands to help you balance on your shoulders as you extend your legs backward, over your head.

If you find it difficult to achieve step 2, break it down into three stages:

1 Raise your legs to an angle of 30° and hold for half a minute before lowering them. When you can hold the position comfortably, practice raising your legs to a 60° angle.

2 When you can hold position 1 comfortably, practice lifting your legs vertically. Hold the position for up to half a minute before lowering them.

3 Now try raising your lower back from the floor (at this stage you will need to tense your leg muscles to raise your legs). When you can hold this position for half a minute, try step 2 again.

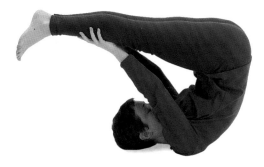

3 When you feel balanced, raise your arms and straighten them, holding onto your shins or, if you can reach, your ankles. Hold the position for as long as you can, closing your eyes and breathing quietly. Imagine yourself floating. When you feel ready, lower your arms and then your legs.

Inversion

························

The plow is one of the great classic positions of yoga. In its first, dynamic, stage, it unwinds the entire spinal column. In the second, static, stage, it encourages the body and mind to achieve a state of pure stillness.

The plow is an asana that takes time and patience to learn and should be carried out slowly and deliberately. Like many classic yoga postures, it offers several variants at increasing levels of difficulty – the choking pose is one – and it needs to be carried out slowly and deliberately, so it can take as long as half an hour from beginning to end.

Because it works on the entire spine, including the network of nerves that emanate from and supply the spinal cord, it is considered one of the most revivifying asanas. It stretches the dorsal (back) muscles, which stimulates the supply of blood to the spinal nerves, so stimulating the entire nervous system. It is even held to have powers of rejuvenation, since it compresses the thyroid gland, whose secretions regu-late the metabolism and act upon the glands. It also compresses the abdomen, which decongests and stimu-lates the organs within it, most beneficially the liver, and including the sexual organs.

The traditional Indian plow gives this pose its name.

This asana should become part of every yoga prac-tice. It is often suggested, however, that it may be used almost as a quick pick-me-up at the end of the day. A minute or two devoted to this posture can revive flag-ging energy in preparation for an active evening, it is claimed. Because the body is in an inverted (upside-down) position during this posture, the blood supply to the head, scalp, and brain is beneficially increased.

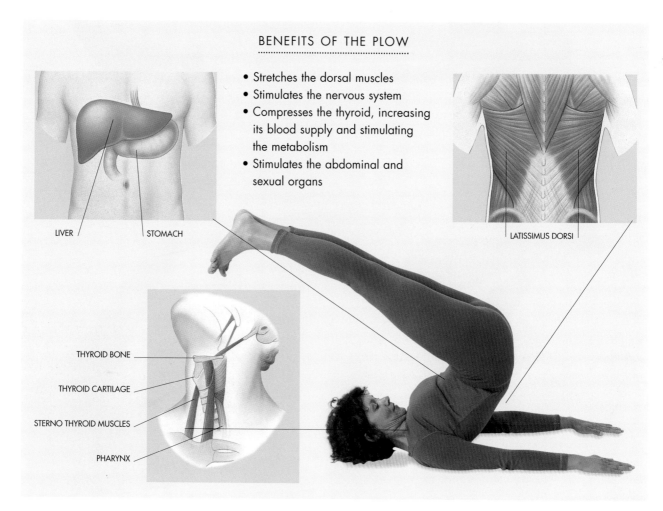

BENEFITS OF THE PLOW
··

- Stretches the dorsal muscles
- Stimulates the nervous system
- Compresses the thyroid, increasing its blood supply and stimulating the metabolism
- Stimulates the abdominal and sexual organs

LIVER STOMACH

LATISSIMUS DORSI

THYROID BONE

THYROID CARTILAGE

STERNO THYROID MUSCLES

PHARYNX

PLOW

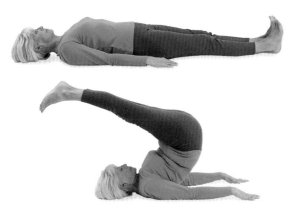

When you feel confident with the pose of tranquility, try moving into the plow. Throughout this posture your breathing should remain normal. In the first stage of the asana you should concentrate on raising your legs in a single, smooth movement and on relaxing all your muscles. In stage 2, you should concentrate on your breathing and on stilling the mind and the body.

CAUTION

If you have breathing difficulties, a hernia, or are suffering nasal congestion do not attempt this exercise.

1 Begin by lying on the floor and follow the first 3 steps of the pose of tranquility sequence described on the previous pages.

2 After performing Step 3, lower your hands from your ankles or shins to the floor and bend your elbows so that your hands lightly support your back. Now lower your legs slowly until your toes touch the floor. Remain calm and relaxed. Hold the position for up to ten breaths, then lower the arms to the floor and use them to maintain balance as you raise your legs and then lower them to the floor.

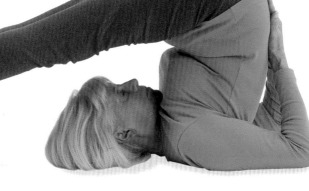

CHOKING POSE

The choking pose is a more advanced version of the plow. If your breathing seems impeded, try breathing more deeply and you will find you can do so.

1 Take up the plow position and hold it for a few seconds, breathing normally. On an out-breath, bend your knees and lower them to the floor in front of your shoulders. Move your arms around to the front and clasp your hands behind your knees beside the crown of your head. Breathe gently and keep the mind quiet.

2 When you are ready, move your hands to the floor behind your back, straighten your legs, then slowly lift them and bring your body back onto the mat.

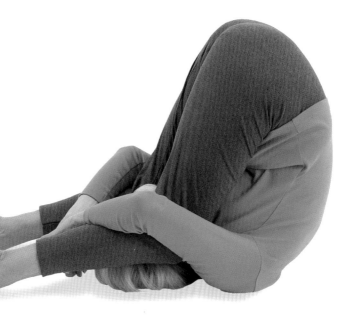

Shoulder Stands

....

Memories of childhood handstands make most students enjoy postures in which they turn upside-down. Shoulder stands are also beneficial to health because they take the pressure off the heart temporarily.

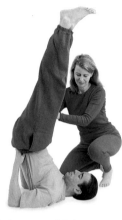

A qualified teacher can help you to attain the shoulder stand.

During a shoulder stand, the chin pressing against the sternum (breast bone) compresses the thyroid gland and increases blood flow to that organ, and stimulates the circulation to the head. For anyone seeking to improve or refine their sense of balance, these inversion postures are absolutely ideal.

Although most people love to do these postures, some are a little nervous about them, often because they are aware that their balance is poor and they are afraid of falling. Yoga can be self-taught, but there are greater benefits in learning from a teacher and attending an evening or weekend course. Any misgivings about falling and other aspects of safety can be dispelled with a skilled teacher to advise and encourage students attempting difficult postures. A teacher will also correct any errors that may have developed with other postures and advise on which postures anyone with particular health problems should avoid and which they should concentrate on. Yoga classes are an ideal way of building confidence in students who approach more acrobatic maneuvers nervously.

These shoulder stands are the first stages in performing head stands, but these should not be attempted without a qualified teacher standing by. Everyone has thoughtlessly balanced on their head when children, but older people are less supple and can injure themselves easily. Pressure on the neck when the head is only slightly misaligned, and falling awkwardly when trying to raise or lower the legs, can result in serious damage to the neck and spine. Anyone suffering from breathing difficulties or pain in the upper spine should not attempt these postures.

HALF-CANDLE

1 *Lie with your head in line with your body, your legs together, feet relaxed, and arms by your sides, palms down. Shake your shoulders slightly to relax them, and lower your chin so that your neck straightens. Breathe out, concentrating on relaxing your whole body.*

During this posture, concentrate on swinging your body smoothly from the floor into the air and back. While you are holding the posture, concentrate on maintaining your balance.

3 *As your legs reach a vertical position, lift your arms and support your trunk with your hands placed in the small of your back. The pressure should be on your shoulders rather than on your neck. Stretch your toes and relax your feet, then hold the position for up to half a minute, breathing slowly and rhythmically.*

2 *Breathe in, and keeping your legs together, swing them upward, followed by your trunk.*

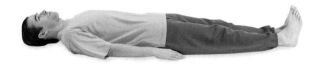

4 *When you are ready, slowly lower your hands onto the mat, then your trunk, followed by your legs. Relax fully for a minute or two.*

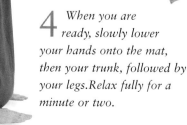

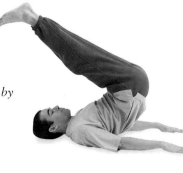

FULL CANDLE

When you are confident with the half-shoulder stand you can move onto the full candle and its variations. In this position your trunk and legs together form an almost vertical line and are at a right angle to your head and shoulders.

CAUTION

If you suffer from heart problems, breathing difficulties or from pain or a slipped disk in the upper spine, do not attempt these postures.

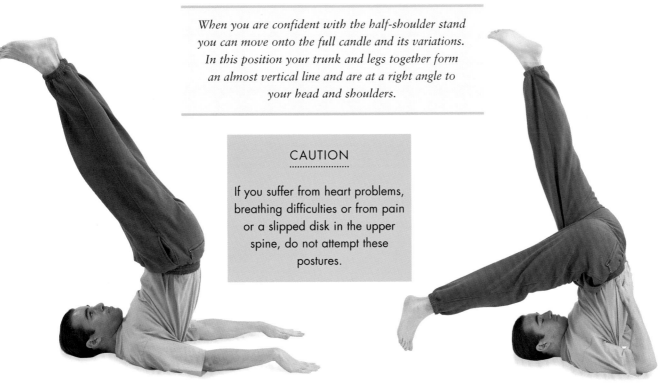

1 *Move into the half-shoulder stand, then lower your hands to help control your balance, straightening your back. Your chin should now press into the hollow called the jugular notch at the top of your sternum (breast bone) and your legs should be straight. After stretching, breathe rhythmically and relax. Hold the position for at least half a minute.*

2 *Assume the full shoulder stand and when you are relaxed lift your hands to support yourself lightly in the small of your back. Breathing out, swing one leg down until your foot touches the floor. Simply let it fall; relax, and let its weight take it down. Now repeat the exercise with the other leg. Repeat before lowering your trunk and your legs to the floor.*

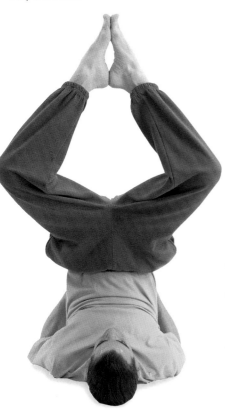

3 *Assume the full shoulder stand and when you are relaxed, support your trunk lightly on your hands. Breathing out, bend your knees outward, breathe in and on the next out-breath bring the soles of your feet together, toes pointing up. Hold the position for a few seconds and on an in-breath, straighten your legs. Repeat the exercise.*

4 *Assume the full shoulder stand, relax, and lift your hands from the floor. Place them against your sides with your palms resting against your thighs. Hold and concentrate on feeling peaceful. When you are ready, lower your arms to the floor to support your trunk as you swing your legs slowly down. Relax.*

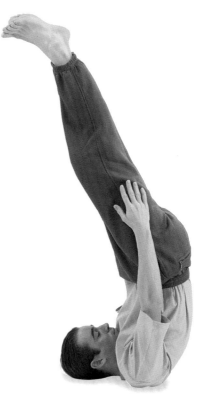

Sun Worship

·······················

Yogis traditionally perform this splendid sequence of exercises at dawn as a prelude to their morning asanas, and in the modern world it makes a perfect start to the day. The exercises originated as a series of devotional movements practiced as a form of worship of the sun.

This corporeal salutation to the dawning of a new day consists of a sequence of 12 stretches, including most forms of movement except for inversion. It can make a good start to a yoga session, toning the muscles and speeding respiration and the heart rate without causing fatigue.

The best approach to Suryanamaskar, the Sanskrit name of the exercises, is to spend some time practicing each exercise separately, trying the easiest ones first. Students who have been working through the stretches and postures described earlier in this section should not find the movements too difficult, and it should take no more than a few days to become familiar with them all.

The next step is to choose a suitable day on which to perform all the exercises in succession. Completing the entire sequence may take a few minutes on the first

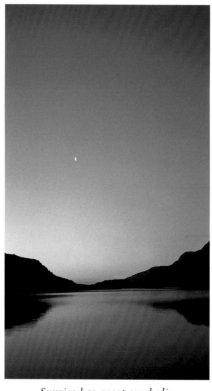

Sunrise has great symbolic importance to yogic practitioners, and many exercises are a form of worship of the sun.

occasion. The salute to the sun is intended to be performed rapidly and rhythmically, however, not slowly. Its purpose is to energize, and students should aim at completing the entire sequence in 20 seconds. Practiced yogis try to work up to repeating the whole salutation 40 times in 10 minutes. To perform the salute to the sun at speed requires a high level of concentration so as to achieve an uninterrupted rhythm. Turn to face the east, think of the invigorating warmth of the sun, and let its cosmic force suffuse your mind and your whole body.

High praise has been heaped on the salute to the sun by converts over the centuries. As well as superb health and vibrant energy, it has been said to rejuvenate, aid weight loss, make the skin glow, release toxins, strengthen the immune system, and even improve the memory.

SALUTE TO THE SUN

Namaste, the prayer position that punctuates many yoga postures, begins and ends the salute to the sun. It is a focus for your concentration at the start of the sequence, and at the end it becomes a pause for relaxation, from which you can go on to a new phase of the day.

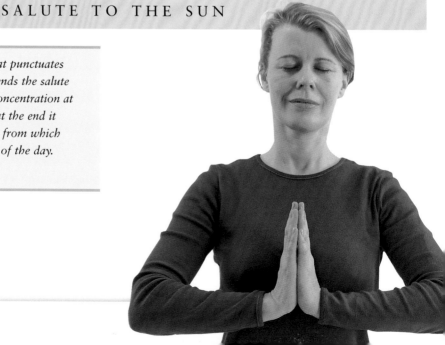

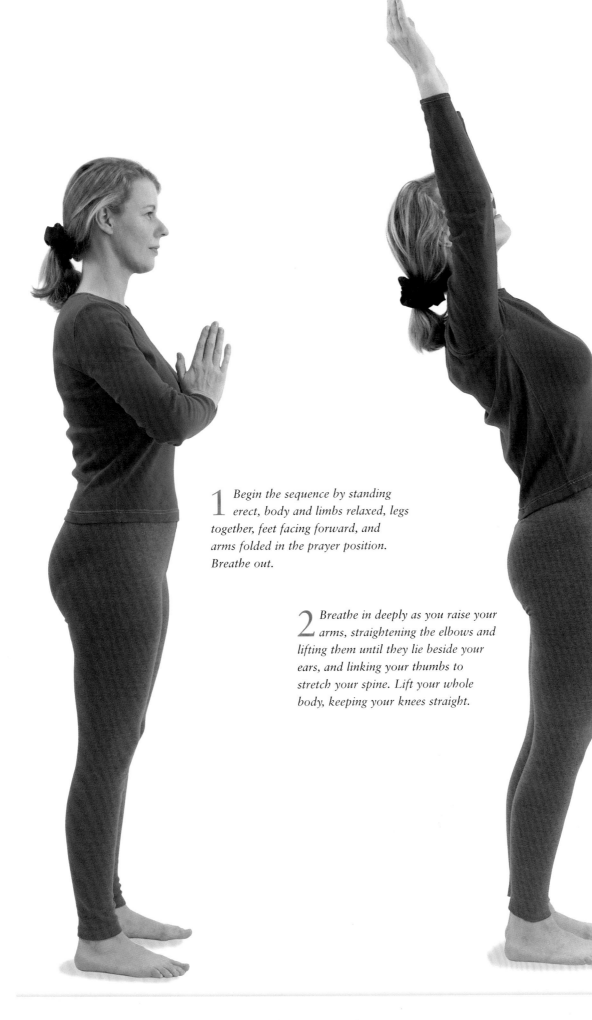

1 Begin the sequence by standing
erect, body and limbs relaxed, legs
together, feet facing forward, and
arms folded in the prayer position.
Breathe out.

2 Breathe in deeply as you raise your
arms, straightening the elbows and
lifting them until they lie beside your
ears, and linking your thumbs to
stretch your spine. Lift your whole
body, keeping your knees straight.

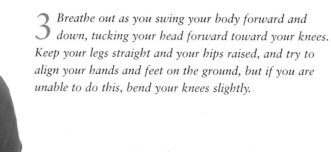

3 Breathe out as you swing your body forward and down, tucking your head forward toward your knees. Keep your legs straight and your hips raised, and try to align your hands and feet on the ground, but if you are unable to do this, bend your knees slightly.

4 Breathe in as in a single movement you raise your trunk, step forward, and bend your right knee, stretching your left leg behind you and placing your hands flat on the floor on either side of your foot, fingers and toes pointing forward. Support yourself on your left foot and right hand. Your right knee is not perpendicular to the floor but bends forward over the foot. Lift up your head.

5 Hold your breath as you pause for an instant, stretching your whole body, then move your right leg back to align it with your left leg and raise your hips and legs clear of the floor, straightening your elbows. Support yourself on your toes and your hands. Do not let your head drop.

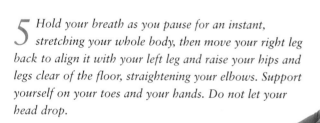

6 Breathe out as you descend to the floor, knees first, followed by the chest, which rests on the floor between your hands, then the forehead or chin. Keep your stomach from resting on the floor.

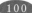

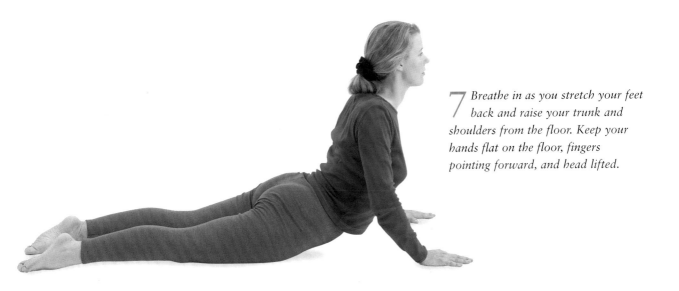

7 Breathe in as you stretch your feet back and raise your trunk and shoulders from the floor. Keep your hands flat on the floor, fingers pointing forward, and head lifted.

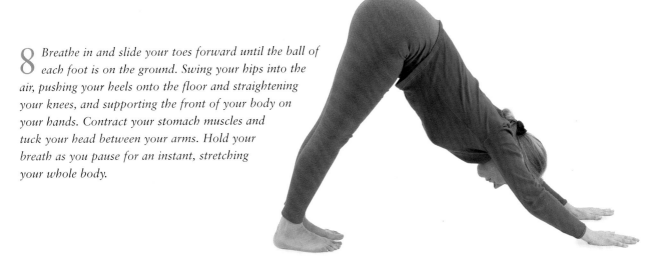

8 Breathe in and slide your toes forward until the ball of each foot is on the ground. Swing your hips into the air, pushing your heels onto the floor and straightening your knees, and supporting the front of your body on your hands. Contract your stomach muscles and tuck your head between your arms. Hold your breath as you pause for an instant, stretching your whole body.

9 Breathe in, move your left foot forward between your hands, and drop your right knee to the floor (the reverse of position 4). Keep your head up. Your legs form an upward-slanting line from right (back) knee to left (front) knee. Hold your breath and pause for an instant, feeling the stretch in your legs.

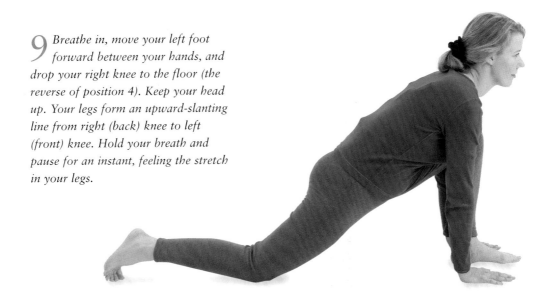

10 Breathe out and keep your hands flat on the floor as you step forward with your right foot to place it beside your left foot and swing your hips up and your trunk forward and down. Keep your hips as high as you can and try to straighten your knees. Tuck your head between your arms.

11 Breathe in deeply as you raise your trunk, your hips, and your arms, reaching forward and up, linking your thumbs above your head and bending the spine backward, as in step 2.

12 Breathe out as you end the sequence by standing erect, arms folded in the prayer position (namaste), elbows out to the sides.

THE PATTERN OF BREATHING DURING THE SALUTE TO THE SUN

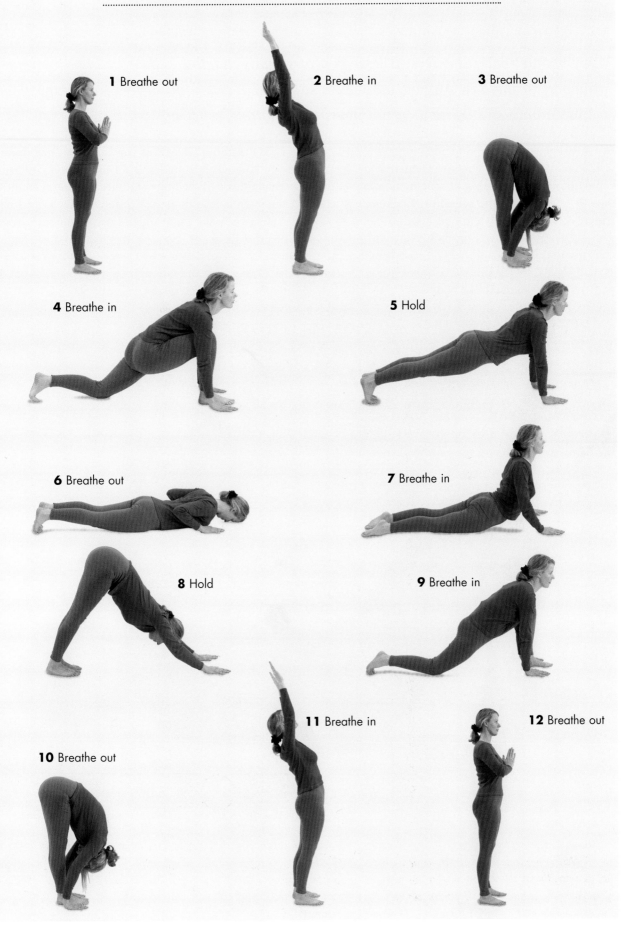

1 Breathe out

2 Breathe in

3 Breathe out

4 Breathe in

5 Hold

6 Breathe out

7 Breathe in

8 Hold

9 Breathe in

10 Breathe out

11 Breathe in

12 Breathe out

The Mudras

·····························

Many people today spend their lives in a physically inactive state – sitting down for a large part of the day. Anyone who leads such a sedentary life suffers from superficial breathing and consequently sluggish circulation, especially to the abdomen.

Massaging the abdominal organs through breathing and other movements speeds up the supply of blood. It also stimulates the motions of the digestive organs and the action of glands such as the pancreas, which supply enzymes used to digest food. This keeps the digestive process healthy and prevents constipation. Abdominal massage also stimulates the sexual organs, which generates feelings of well-being and vitality in the mind and body.

The mudras are a set of yoga exercises that imitate body language. A mudra is an expression of energy moving through the body and there are many mudras, each intended to stimulate a different part of the body.

Exercises like these address one of the most widespread causes of poor body image: a distended stomach. These progressive exercises, carried out regularly, tone up and strengthen the muscles of the abdomen, buttocks, thighs, and calves.

ASWINI MUDRA

This simple mudra exercises the pelvic muscles that control the opening of the rectum and bladder, so helping to prevent incontinence. It is particularly important for women since it strengthens the pelvic floor muscles, preventing prolapse of the uterus.

THE FEMALE PELVIC REGION
·····························

UTERUS — — BLADDER

RECTUM — — URETHRA

PELVIC FLOOR — — VAGINA

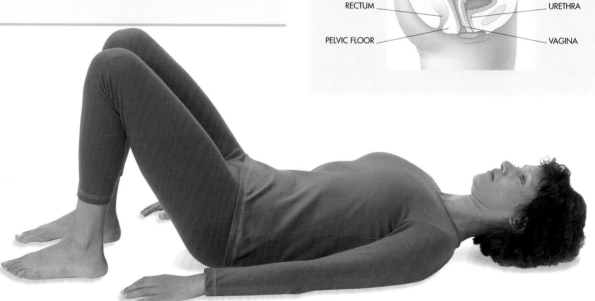

1 *Lie on your back and bend your knees, drawing your heels toward your hips. Breathe rhythmically for a few minutes. Contract the sphincter muscle (at the opening of your rectum) and relax it two or three times. Women should simultaneously contract and relax the muscles of the vagina.*

2 *Next, pull the sphincter muscle and all the muscles of your pelvis inward and upward, and relax them. Practice contracting and relaxing all your pelvic muscles two or three times, then try to do it in time with your breathing. Practice this for up to half a minute, then relax.*

3 *Practice step 2 every day until you can contract and relax your muscles rhythmically for five minutes. Then try doing the exercise in a kneeling position, sitting, or standing, and independently of your breathing rhythm.*

YOGA MUDRA

To practice this asana effectively it is important to keep your buttocks firmly against your heels and not to lift them when stretching your spine forward. If your back is not very supple, you will find this impossible at first, but with daily practice preceded by relaxed breathing you will eventually be able to bend a little further forward each day until you can touch the ground with your forehead, the tip of your nose, and your chin. Breathing is not impeded by the posture and you should be able to work up to holding it for up to ten minutes. It improves the functioning of the liver, spleen, kidneys, pancreas, bladder, and uterus, and relieves constipation.

THE ABDOMINAL ORGANS

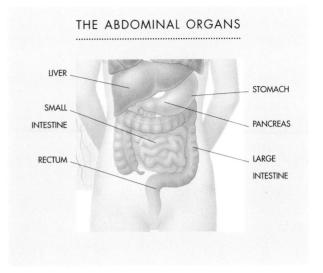

LIVER

STOMACH

SMALL
INTESTINE

PANCREAS

RECTUM

LARGE
INTESTINE

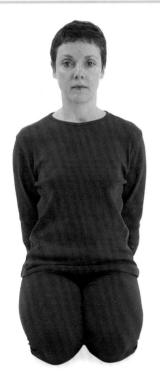

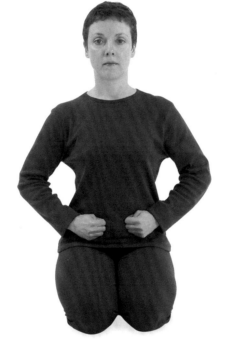

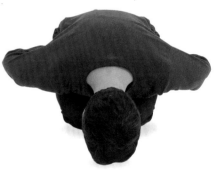

1 *Kneel on the mat and sit back on your heels. Your trunk should be erect and your head balanced. Place your hands, palms down, on your heels. Breathe out.*

2 *On the in-breath, raise your hands to waist level, fold your fingers over your thumbs to make a fist, and place a fist either side of your navel.*

3 *Breathe out, stretch your spine, and, while keeping your buttocks resting firmly on your ankles, slowly bend your body above the waist forward as far as you can. Hold the position, breathing normally and concentrating on relaxing your muscles, for at least a minute. Then sit back on your heels, rest your hands on your thighs, and relax for a minute or two.*

CAUTION

If you are pregnant, or suffer from hernias or other abdominal complaints, do not attempt this exercise.

The Bandhas

....

The Sanskrit word bandha means "lock" or "contraction," and in the context of yoga it describes blocking the out-breath temporarily. Generations ago, yogis discovered that blocking the passage of air through the lungs temporarily is an excellent way of stimulating the abdominal organs.

Uddiyana bandha is one of the most spectacular postures of yoga. The entire stomach seems to disappear, leaving a large hollow below the rib cage. In its full classic form it causes the transverse muscles of the abdomen, the external oblique muscles, which normally compress the contents of the abdomen, to stand out very prominently. This is difficult, however, and is achieved in the advanced form of the posture.

The purpose of this asana is to massage the organs of the chest and abdomen. It mimics the up-and-down motion of the diaphragm, massaging the heart and restoring the diaphragm's elasticity. Exercising the lungs when the amount of air they contain is reduced helps strengthen them. The exercise pulls the stomach up toward the rib cage, invigorating the blood supply to the abdominal organs and stimulating the digestive system. It also acts on the solar plexus, which transmits impulses between the brain and the abdominal organs, regularizing the activity of the nerves.

The bandhas are classic yoga postures, and act as a tonic for minor physical illnesses and as a form of preventive medicine that benefits the whole body.

UDDIYANA BANDHA

For this exercise to be effective you must not have eaten for at least four hours. You must also make sure that you breathe out as much air as you can, and that you do not breathe in again until the very end of the exercise, when your stomach is in its normal position, or you might damage your lungs.

1 *Stand with your feet a shoulder's width apart and parallel to each other. Stoop down so that your back is slightly rounded and your knees bent a little. Place your hands on your thighs with your thumbs closest to your groin. Contract your neck and shoulders and push your elbows forward, to enable your arms to support your shoulders during the exercise.*

2 *Breathe out forcefully and simultaneously contract the muscles of your abdomen so that your lungs are emptied of as much air as possible.*

3 *Without breathing in, quickly relax your abdominal muscles and expand your rib cage as if you were breathing deeply. When you do this, your ribs will rise and your diaphragm will move up, causing your stomach to move inward. Hold the position for about five seconds.*

4 *Let the rib cage and the stomach return to their normal position, then breathe in. Air will enter your lungs quite gently. Stand erect and breathe normally for a few minutes.*

CAUTION

....

If you are menstruating or pregnant or suffer from heart disease, breathing disorders, or any disorder of the abdominal organs, do not attempt this exercise.

YONIMUDRA AND NADABANDA

Several bandhas and the mudras (see pages 104–105) complement each other, and some are used as aids to meditation, as this example shows. Yonimudra is a classic asana that stimulates the nerves of the face and the skull. However, performed correctly it also causes a ringing sound, called the nada, to fill the ears. By concentrating totally on this sound – the technique called nadabanda – it is possible to ascend to a higher state of meditation.

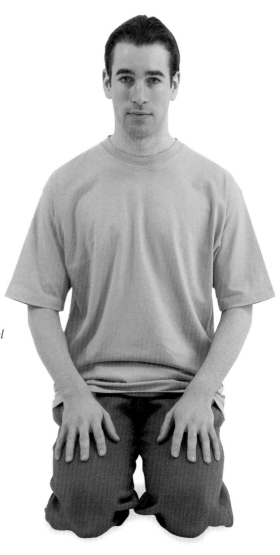

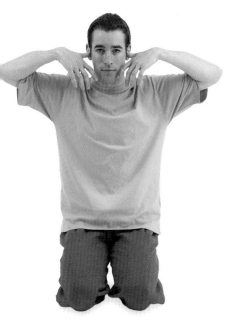

1 *Sit erect on the floor on your heels or with your legs crossed and your hands resting on your knees. Raise your hands level with your face and your elbows to shoulder level.*

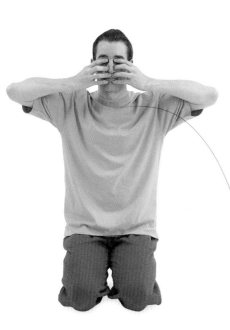

2 *Insert your thumbs in your ears and press slightly to cut out external sounds. Close your eyes and place your index fingers across your eyelids, pressing gently on the lower part of the eyeball. Breathe in and hold your breath, placing your middle fingers on either side of your nose. Place your third fingers above your upper lip and your fourth fingers beneath your lower lip, and press them together to close your lips. You should hear a low ringing sound inside your head. Concentrate on this sound, called the nada, for about half a minute, then release your fingers and breathe normally.*

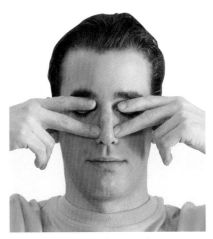

3 *Repeat step 2 three or four times, holding your breath a little longer each time, trying to concentrate totally on the nada sound, which should increase as your concentration intensifies.*

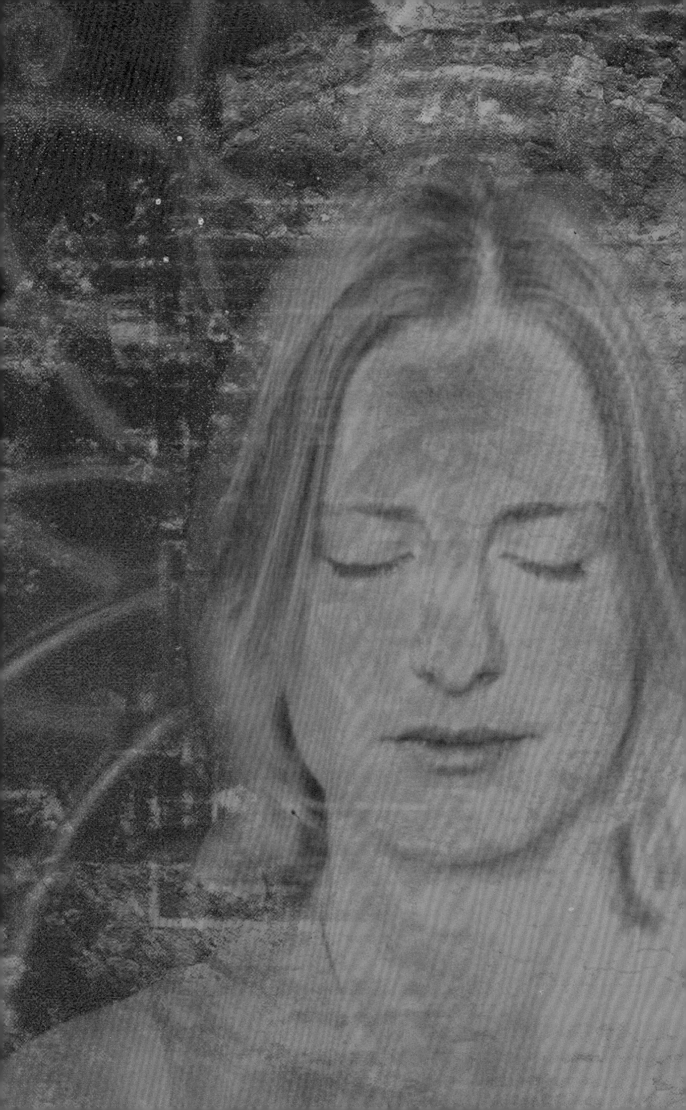

Part Seven

Breathing
Techniques

Special Breathing Techniques

···

*Once effective breathing has become second nature it may be
time to learn some techniques designed especially to benefit
certain body systems and organs. There are exercises to clear the
entire respiratory system of the effects of pollution, and rhythmic
breathing patterns that produce soporific humming sounds.
And kumbhaka – the technique of restraining the breath – is a
powerful stimulus to mental concentration.*

Only when beginners are confident that their breathing is effective (see pages 52–57) should they try any of the special breathing techniques illustrated in this chapter, and anyone whose respiration has been affected by illness must allow several weeks of remedial breathing practice. The asana on page 112, shining head, stimulates the nervous system by vigorous breathing through the nose several times in succession. This cleansing process makes breathing easier and more effective and the head, brain, and nervous system benefit from better blood circulation. Bellows breath (see page 112) energizes the body and stimulates the liver, spleen, and pancreas so these organs function more efficiently, improving digestion.

People living where air quality is poor, former smokers, and people with asthma can benefit from lung-clearing exercises (see page 113). Worsening air quality worldwide makes it important to breathe through the nose and not through the mouth. As air is drawn through the nose, along the windpipe and into the lungs, it is warmed by the body's heat, and minute, mucus-covered hairs lining the nostrils trap particles which might damage the lungs.

In these cleansing exercises breathing must not be silent. In bellows breath, for instance air is drawn into the nostrils and forced out very audibly. Some asanas, however, involve making sounds like humming, deep in the throat (see pages 116-7). This is hard to learn, but enjoyable, and it induces calm and peace of mind.

Breathing is controlled by the unconscious, but the conscious influences breathing rate and depth, so we can breathe faster when we exercise, for example. Only during emergencies does the brain override the will – when we are in danger and a decision that affects survival becomes imperative. Then breathing stops for an instant. This concentrates the mind totally for the few seconds needed to decide and take action. This reaction, imitated in yoga in a technique known as kumbhaka or holding the breath (see pages 118-9), is an effective way of focusing the mind.

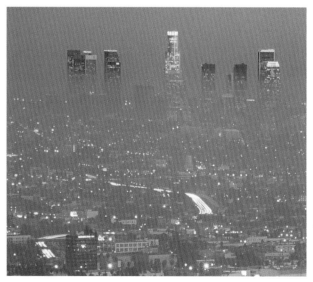

*Breathing through the nose helps reduce the effects
of atmospheric pollution in modern cities.*

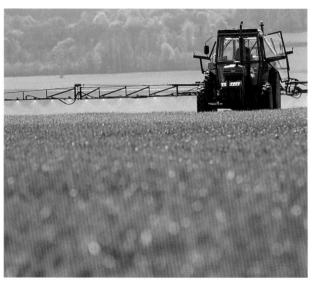

*Intensive farming, which involves the spraying of crops,
pollutes the air in the countryside.*

BENEFITS OF SPECIAL BREATHING TECHNIQUES

People who must endure poor air quality for prolonged periods can benefit from the asanas on the following pages. Some cleanse the lungs and air passages, while others stimulate the brain and nervous system and eliminate diseases from the head.

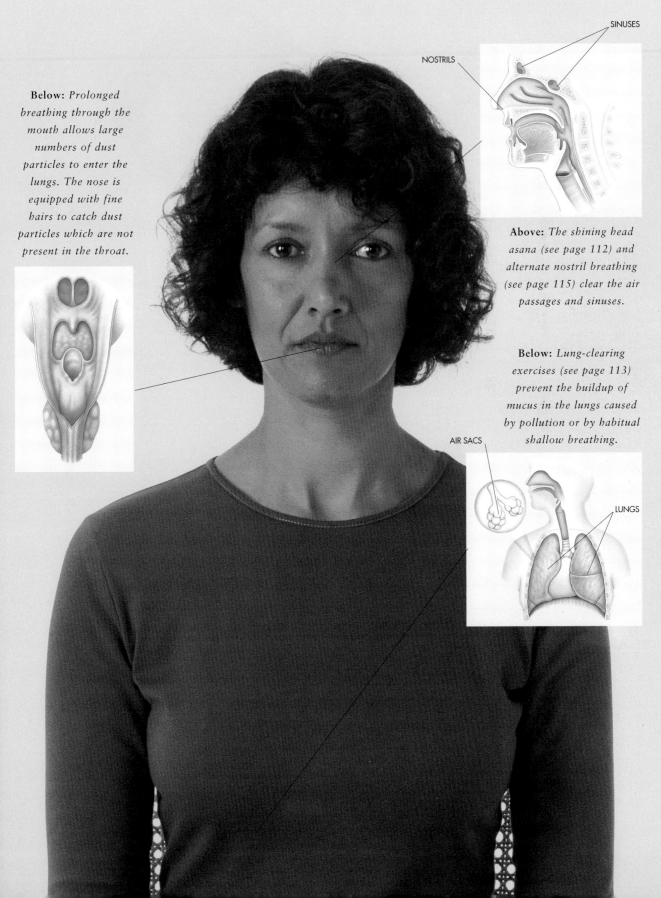

Below: *Prolonged breathing through the mouth allows large numbers of dust particles to enter the lungs. The nose is equipped with fine hairs to catch dust particles which are not present in the throat.*

SINUSES

NOSTRILS

Above: *The shining head asana (see page 112) and alternate nostril breathing (see page 115) clear the air passages and sinuses.*

Below: *Lung-clearing exercises (see page 113) prevent the buildup of mucus in the lungs caused by pollution or by habitual shallow breathing.*

AIR SACS

LUNGS

SHINING HEAD

The immediate effect of this exercise is to clear the nostrils and the sinuses. Breathing becomes easier and more effective and the head, brain, and nervous system benefit from the increased efficiency of blood circulation which results.

1 *Stand erect or sit on the heels. Lean the trunk forward and place your hands on your thighs.*

2 *Breathe in quite gently through the nose, then breathe out quickly and forcefully through the nose, pulling in your abdominal muscles strongly as you do so. Breathe in and out in this way 10–12 times in succession, concentrating on expelling in every out-breath all the pollutants and impurities your body has been breathing in.*

3 *Stop if you feel giddy; close your eyes and breathe normally until the feeling has passed. Perform step 2 once on the first occasion, but work cautiously up to repeating the exercise two or three times in a session for the greatest therapeutic value.*

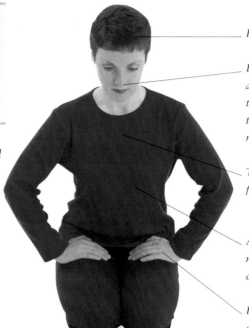

— Head balanced

— Breathing in and out through the nose, not through the mouth

— Trunk leaning forward

— Abdominal muscles contracted

— Hands resting on the thighs

BELLOWS BREATH

Out-breaths

During step 1, contract your abdominal muscles as you breathe out to force the air out of your lungs. Keep your head erect and concentrate on the air clearing your frontal sinuses as it flows audibly out through your open nostrils. The slow out-breath during step 2 should be less forceful.

Bellows breath blasts the body with energy. It is important in these cleansing exercises not to try to breathe silently, as in relaxed breathing; air should be drawn into the nostrils and forced out audibly, so that it sounds like a bellows or, in Sanskrit, a bhastrika.

In-breaths

During step 1, make the in-breaths as forcible and audible as the out-breaths, keeping your head up. Your diaphragm should move and your lungs inflate, but not your abdomen. The long in-breath during step 2 should be slower and less forceful.

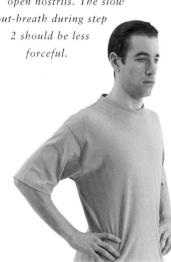

1 *Stand erect, feet apart, then lean forward and place your hands on your hips. Breathe in and out rapidly and forcefully through both nostrils 10–12 times in succession, maintaining an even breathing rhythm.*

2 *After the 12th out-breath, stop, take a deep, slow in-breath, pressing your chin into your chest. Hold your breath for as long as you can, then raise your head and breathe out slowly and completely.*

3 *Stop immediately if you feel dizzy; close your eyes, and breathe normally until the feeling has passed.*

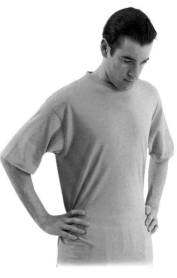

LUNG-CLEARING EXERCISE

This exercise is especially beneficial to people living in the world's growing and increasingly polluted cities, and in rural areas where crops are sprayed, since it compresses the lungs and massages them, causing dirt and impurities to be dislodged and expelled. You should attempt this exercise only if your lungs are healthy, however. If you have bronchitis, emphysema, or you experience chest pains do not attempt it.

Head upright

Shoulders relaxed

Elbows well back

Abdomen relaxed

1 *Stand erect with your feet apart and your arms by your sides. Breathe out, and on the in-breath raise your arms and hands, palm upward, level with your shoulders. Bend your elbows and rest the tips of your fingers on your shoulder joints.*

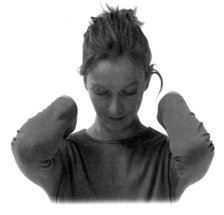

2 *Holding your breath, let your head fall forward until your chin touches your chest. Then, move your elbows forward, putting pressure on your chest. Continue holding your breath for a few seconds more. Then breathe out, raise your head, and move your elbows in line with your shoulders. Straighten your arms and lower them to your sides. Repeat the exercise three or four times.*

Feet a shoulder width apart

CAUTION

If you have high blood pressure or suffer from serious chest complaints, such as chronic bronchitis, asthma, or emphysema, do not attempt these exercises.

Alternate Nostril Breathing

To practice breathing through alternate nostrils is an important step in mastering breath control, and it ensures that the body's energy needs and supplies are kept in balance. It has recently been discovered that breathing through one nostril stimulates the opposite hemisphere of the brain, so when the right side of the brain becomes active, the breathing changes to the left nostril, and vice versa.

Although we are unaware of it, we breathe through both nostrils equally only for about 20 percent of the time. Among the most common reasons is a blockage in the sinuses – the air-filled spaces in the bones around the nose, which cause the voice to resonate. For centuries, yogis have understood that keeping both nostrils fully functioning is essential to maintain effective mental activity. However, only now has medical research confirmed that we breathe naturally through alternate nostrils. Developing the habits of breathing through the nose, and of keeping the nostrils and sinuses clear, is important to health.

A group of the many energy-expanding yoga techniques called pranayamas focuses on controlling the breath for a number of different health reasons. The earliest and most basic of these techniques, with the simple, descriptive name of "alternate nostril breath," ensures that each nostril functions fully and effectively. Since the air that enters the body through the nose is cleansed and warmed, the body benefits if we develop the habit of breathing through the nose for most of the time. It is really only necessary to breathe through the mouth when more air than usual is needed for running or exercising very vigorously.

CLOSING THE NOSTRILS

In yoga, the following technique is used to close the nostrils. It closes each nostril completely while reducing necessary movement of the hand to a minimum so that concentration is not interrupted.

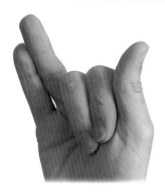

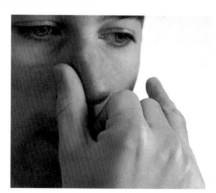

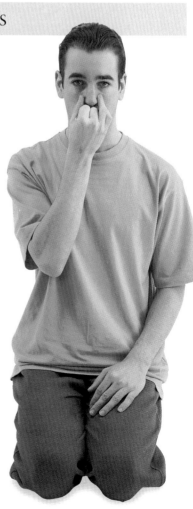

1 *Bend the first and second fingers of your right hand, leaving the third and fourth fingers extended; rest your thumb against the folded first finger.*

2 *With the inside of your hand toward your face, press the inside of the extended right thumb against your right nostril to close it.*

3 *Use the same hand to close the left nostril by pressing the extended third finger against it.*

ALTERNATE NOSTRIL BREATH

This exercise helps clear the nostrils so that they can both function properly. Repeat the exercise up to five times maximum the first time you do it, then in subsequent sessions gradually build up to about 12 repetitions.

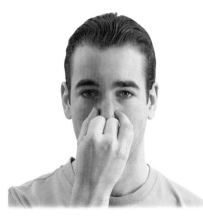

1 *Close your right nostril with your thumb and, keeping it closed, breathe in through the left nostril, counting up to four.*

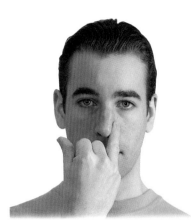

2 *Hold your breath and count to 16, while opening the right nostril and closing the left with your third finger.*

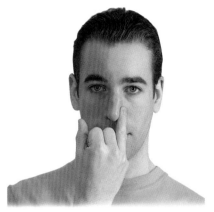

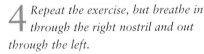

3 *Breathe out slowly through the right nostril to a count of 8.*

4 *Repeat the exercise, but breathe in through the right nostril and out through the left.*

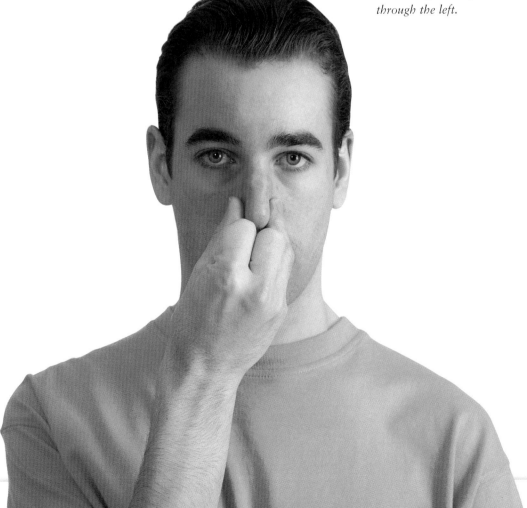

115

Making Sounds

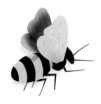

The sound of a buzzing bee is the effect in bhramari.

Although normal breathing should be almost silent, respiration and making sounds are inseparable bodily processes. Chanting and singing involve vigorous, controlled breathing and are natural to people everywhere. Midway between audible breathing and chanting is humming. It is melodious and rhythmical, and it sets up a pleasant vibration that can be felt through the body.

The pranayamas are breathing techniques for increasing energy. Bhastrika or bellows breath on page 112 is one. Another, *sitkari* on page 149, is a cooling technique that relieves fatigue caused by heat. Bhramari – the Sanskrit word for bee – is one of several pranayamas that make sounds. When performed correctly the noise produced is like a contented snoring or a bee buzzing.

These "sounding breaths" are sometimes difficult at first. It is worth persevering, however, because their long-term effects are extremely beneficial. *Ujjaii*, shown opposite, is an ancient technique which will eventually lower the blood pressure, and, it is claimed, can overcome all diseases. It is believed to keep illness at bay by cleansing and toning the whole body, and it does this by increasing the amount of oxygen inhaled.

BLACK BEE

This is a good exercise just before bedtime if you find it difficult to sleep, since you concentrate on the relaxing, almost hypnotic effect of the sounds you produce. Perhaps because it is so relaxing it is also a good asana to do at the end of a hard day's work, so that you will feel energized and ready to go on with your evening schedule.

GOOD VIBRATIONS

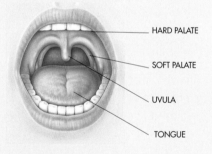

HARD PALATE

SOFT PALATE

UVULA

TONGUE

1 *Sit cross-legged on the floor, or stand with your feet a shoulder width apart, erect but relaxed. Take a deep, slow in-breath through the nose and hold your breath for a few seconds.*

2 *Open your mouth and breathe out slowly through the mouth, not the nose, making a low "ung" sound as you do so. Practice until you can extend the "ung" sound into a low humming, and you can feel vibrations.*

3 *Repeat steps 1 and 2, holding your breath for as long as you can at the end of step 1, focusing on the rhythmic hum and the pleasing vibrations through your body.*

The vibrations on breathing in are caused by the soft palate being drawn up toward the wall of the throat. As you breathe out, the soft palate descends and the uvula, which is composed of muscle and mucous membrane, vibrates.

Head upright and balanced, eyes facing forward

Shoulders relaxed

Trunk upright

Hands relaxed, resting on the knees

UJJAII

In this exercise you make a sound rather like a long drawn-out sob while breathing in and breathing out. To do this you have to half-close the glottis (the part of the larynx that contains the vocal cords and the slitlike opening that lies between them). This may take some practice. Try tensing the muscle of the throat and breathing out to produce a roaring sound. It is easy to breathe out too forcefully at first, so once you can produce a roar, try roaring more gently. Then work at prolonging the roar until you can produce a sound rather more like a controlled moan.

CAUTION

If you suffer from breathing problems, approach these exercises with care. Stop if they cause discomfort or dizziness and consult a physician. If you suffer from emphysema do not attempt them.

THE THROAT

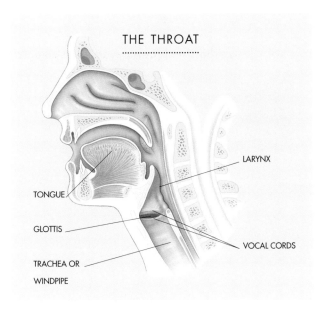

TONGUE

GLOTTIS

TRACHEA OR
WINDPIPE

LARYNX

VOCAL CORDS

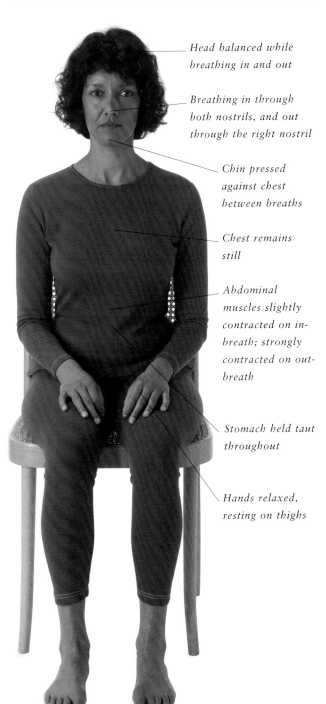

Head balanced while breathing in and out

Breathing in through both nostrils, and out through the right nostril

Chin pressed against chest between breaths

Chest remains still

Abdominal muscles slightly contracted on in-breath; strongly contracted on out-breath

Stomach held taut throughout

Hands relaxed, resting on thighs

1 Stand or sit with the trunk erect but comfortable. Close your mouth and breathe in through both nostrils at once, partially closing off the glottis, and contracting the muscles of the abdomen slightly. Practice doing this until you produce a hum which can be felt as a vibration in the throat, not from the nose.

2 Partially close the glottis, raise your right hand and close your right nostril (see page 115). Breathe out more slowly through the left nostril. Again, you should produce a continuous sound, something like a sob or a moan.

3 Practice steps 1–4 three or four times at first, working up to 12 repetitions in three minutes.

4 When you feel experienced, let your chin drop to your chest after step 1, and hold your breath for as long as you can, working to hold it four times as long as you took to breathe in.

Breath Retention

Breath retention (holding the breath) is one of many yoga techniques that developed because, centuries ago, yogis tried to imitate the actions of the body. They discovered that stopping the breath for a short time, a technique they called kumbhaka, could be a useful way of concentrating the mind. They found that interrupting the breathing before inhalation is especially beneficial because it tranquilizes the mind, bringing about the state of calm that must precede meditation.

Breathing can also be stopped before exhaling, and, indeed, during exhalation and inhalation. Yoga teaches all four as techniques for exercising control over the mind. Beginners can usually hold their breath in for only a short time but in time they learn to prolong this to two minutes, benefiting from the restful feeling it brings. "The human body" writes Swami Kuvalayananda, "is constantly at work even when it is apparently at rest ... Engines built by humans can be switched off to minimize wear and tear and overheating. We cannot switch off our engines without dying, but we can let them idle and see that they are properly maintained."

Pauses in breathing represent the nearest humans get to stillness. Not only do they heighten the ability to concentrate but they also deepen the sense of voluntary control over the life force and through it over one's own life.

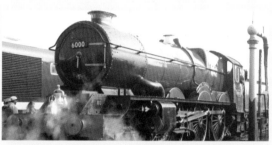

In kumbhaka, the vibration in the body is like that of a locomotive stationary under steam, its driver alert and ready to start, but relaxed. Similarly, the prana [Life Force] vibrates in the torso, but the consciousness is kept relaxed and ready to let go or let in the breath.

B.K.S. Iyengar, *Light on Yoga*

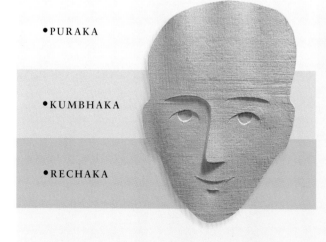

•PURAKA

•KUMBHAKA

•RECHAKA

Yoga teaches that all the rhythmic cycles of the universe are composed of puraka, kumbhaka, and rechaka. As long as the rhythmic breathing cycle continues, we live in the body.

THE THREE PHASES OF BREATHING

The pranayama or life force is said to flow through the breath, which has three phases:

- puraka—inhalation

- kumbhaka—retention or pause

- rechaka—exhalation

Each in-breath is the next moment of life. Tension and depression restrict and deplete puraka and inhibit rechaka, the state of "giving back." One of the effects of kumbhaka is to concentrate the mind, which relieves tension and restores tranquility.

RESTRAINING THE BREATH

Practice kumbhaka only when you have been practicing effective natural breathing for some time. At first, you may be able to hold your breath in for only half a minute. You may also feel slightly giddy, although this should fade quickly. If it persists, breathe out, relax, and do not practice kumbhaka again before consulting a physician. By practicing two or three times a week, you will gain control over your breathing and be able to hold your breath for up to two minutes.

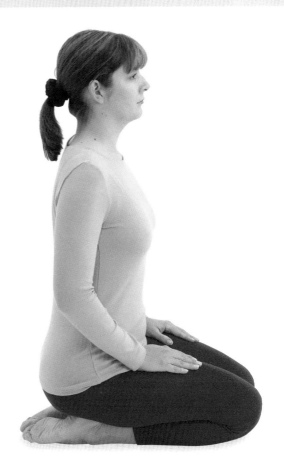

1 *Kneel on the floor and sink back on your heels. Your back should be erect and your head balanced. Place your hands on your thighs. Breathe in and out for a few minutes and concentrate on relaxing.*

2 *Breathe out and then breathe in deeply and slowly. Drop your chin to your chest and rest it on the jugular notch.*

3 *Hold your breath. Concentrate on relaxing first your abdominal muscles and then any other tense muscles. Your trunk should feel light, as though you are sitting on a cushion of air. Do not worry about your breathing. Concentrate instead on feeling still. Think about peace and calm.*

4 *Signals from your brain will urge you to breathe out and take another breath. When they become too strong to ignore, lift your head and breathe gently out. Then breathe normally for two or three minutes.*

5 *Repeat steps 2–4 two or three times, then breathe normally and relax.*

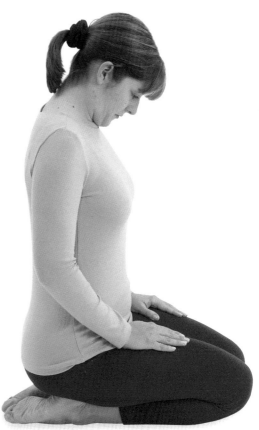

CAUTION
....

If you suffer from chest or heart problems or hypertension do not practice kumbhaka.

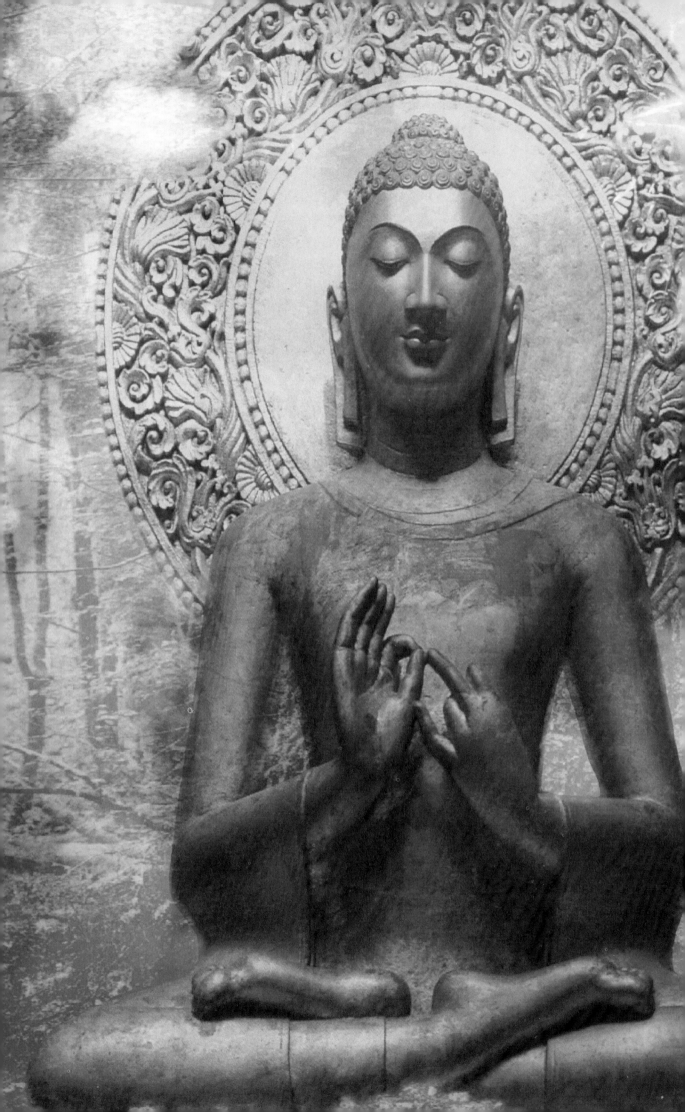

Part Eight

Meditation

··

The Way to Meditation

For many thousands of years meditation has been central to the development and practice of yoga. Only during the 20th century have schools of yoga emerged that ignore the mind and focus exclusively on exercising the body. Hatha yoga bridges the gap between traditional and new approaches, teaching ways of concentrating and controlling the mind alongside stretching exercises and asanas.

Some people who practice yoga in the West today try to reject all mental aspects of yoga, and devote themselves instead to learning and perfecting asanas – the physical side alone. That is not really yoga, but a form of gymnastics. To alleviate illness and maintain health, to overcome mental problems, and sustain a sense of calm and well-being involves an interplay between mind and body. To develop the body without involving the mind is possible – just as it is possible to learn to do every posture in this book without learning how to be calm, fulfilled, or happy.

There are many yogis who follow the paths of the classic yoga schools of meditation, seeking to achieve a mystical state of union with the universe. But most people who practice meditation do so for simpler reasons, to overcome feelings of dissatisfaction and to develop a more serene outlook.

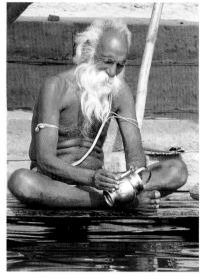

Wandering Hindu holy men, sadhus, still live ascetic lives in India, practicing yoga and meditation.

In essence, yoga is meditation. *The Yoga Sutras*, the second-century BCE writings of the sage Patañjali, is a collection of meditations. The yoga sages practiced few asanas other than cross-legged sitting positions in which they could sit without moving for long periods. Achieving the concentration necessary to meditation can be difficult, however. About 1,000 years ago hatha yoga developed to complement the classic approaches by offering physical techniques such as deep breathing and the practice of asanas. The object of these techniques is to deepen concentration in preparation for meditation.

People who are just beginning hatha yoga often find themselves dismayed at the prospect of trying to govern their emotions and control their racing thoughts, and prefer to concentrate on stretching and exercise. Gradually, however, through deep breathing and relaxation, they find themselves gaining control over the mind without even trying. Many hatha yoga teachers encourage their strengthening confidence by introducing them to simple meditation techniques very early on. When they are making progress with the asanas and have practiced rhythmic breathing, students are encouraged to improve their concentration by practicing visualization (focusing the mind on an image with positive associations) while practicing the asanas. Later, they may begin short sessions aimed at focusing the mind and improving concentration, perhaps with the help of chanting or other techniques (see page 131).

Learning how to avoid being overwhelmed by the senses is the first stage on the way to acquiring the dispassionate outlook that is necessary to acquire full control of the mind. The following eight pages explore ways of learning to control the mind, which may lead eventually to practicing deeper meditation.

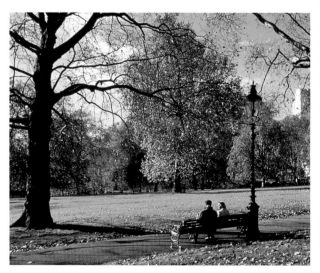

Contemplating the beauty of nature is a simple way of learning to focus the mind.

THE ESSENTIAL ASPECTS OF MEDITATION

ASANAS

Through the asanas you gain control over the body and develop the ability to be still. Being able to remain without moving for long periods is a meditation technique.

ALTERING AWARENESS

The philosophy of yoga encourages a dispassionate attitude that enables you to experience a different and often more satisfying reality than the one constantly glimpsed through overwhelming emotion.

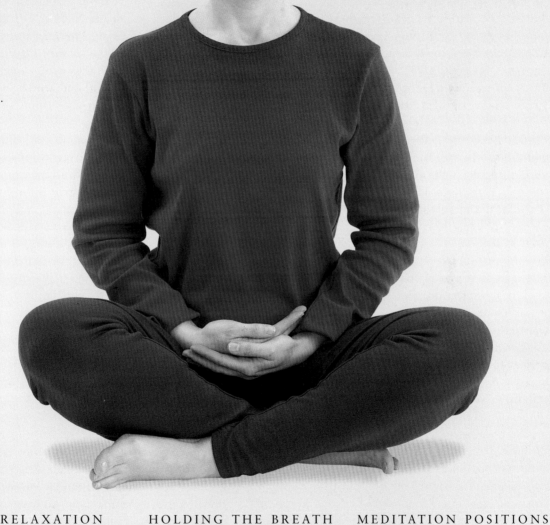

DEEP RELAXATION

Learning to relax the body and the mind is a way of exercising mental control. Being able to relax at will helps the mind to see beyond the intensity of minor frustrations in daily life.

HOLDING THE BREATH

In hatha yoga, breathing is an important preparation for meditation, for breathing techniques teach an aspect of mental control. Gradually bringing the mind under the control of the will encourages greater awareness, which is one way of expanding consciousness.

MEDITATION POSITIONS

It is possible to meditate in any position – sitting in a chair or on the floor, even standing. The Buddha is traditionally depicted practicing yoga: sitting meditating in the lotus position – cross-legged, with each foot resting, sole upward, on the opposite thigh.

Mind Control

························

Remembering to stand upright instead of just standing up is a sign that the mind is beginning to take control. So is thinking about doing some yoga practice at the same time on two successive days. And occasionally, stopping dead, switching off, and just breathing for a while instead of getting worked up about something is evidence that the mind is winning the battle against uncontrolled emotions.

The idea of having to learn to control the mind can be a hurdle to people thinking of taking up yoga. Perhaps they imagine themselves painfully forcing creaking knees into the lotus position, and struggling to think about cosmic forces for hours on end while trying not to wriggle. They cannot see themselves ever succeeding. But for 1,000 years or more teachers of hatha yoga have been instructing beginners in the basics of meditation and mind control. They know that neither the body nor the mind can be forced into doing anything that it does not want to do. Hatha yoga is taught in ways that are so subtle and integrated that students often think they are learning something else.

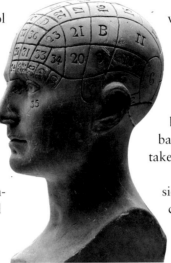

The mind is a mystery, but yoga teaches ways to explore it and unlock some of its secrets.

ways friends speak about each other as their moods change and as events in their lives unfold. Learning to control mental activities means learning not to allow sensory impressions to dominate, so that events and situations can be seen in their true light, and to hold back calmly when emotions threaten to take over.

While teachers introduce short sessions focusing on concentration into their classes, students teaching themselves sometimes find it difficult to begin. If "I can't do that" is the first response, it is worth considering that simply sitting for a few minutes, breathing rhythmically, and working on adopting a positive attitude could be a valuable first session. Reflect

Yoga teaches control of the mind gently. The emphasis in the asanas is on easing the body into positions that seem impossible at first. Just sitting on the heels will be difficult for a beginner who for years has sat only on chairs and exercised very little. But, constantly reassured that it will eventually happen, taught to relax and to breathe rhymically for greater flexibility, the beginner practices every day and is sitting on the heels within a week. Given time, the most difficult asana can be mastered by the same method. These two techniques – using the power of the breath to work on the interrelationship between mind and body, and improving physical flexibility – work together to bring about mental control. And by increasing control over the mind students find their breathing improves, they can relax more effectively, and perform the asanas more easily.

Mastering mind control helps people manage their lives more effectively. "When not controlling his thoughts" wrote Patañjali in the *The Yoga Sutras*, "a man remains their slave." Memory and sensory impressions are unreliable – think of the different

that controlling the mind is a natural process, and if it seems difficult, overcoming difficulties is part of being human. Making a commitment to devote time each week to breathing, relaxing, and feeling calm is a step on the path to meditation.

Through its long history, yoga has repeatedly advanced our understanding of the power of the mind. For example, it has revealed that the mind can be harnessed to speed the healing of injuries. During the early 1980s an experiment was carried out at the Yoga for Health Foundation in England to measure the electrical receptivity of the tissue fluid around a fractured cheekbone. The fluid's receptivity was found to be much lower than in undamaged parts of the body. After five minutes of breathing deeply and imagining electromagnetic energy flowing into the fractured bone, the injured person was tested for a second time and the electrical receptivity of the area around it was found to equal that outside it.

There are many techniques of mind control. The injured person in this experiment used visualization, a technique that is explored on the following pages.

OVERCOMING INHIBITIONS

The ability to control the mind is innate. Babies learn to walk without the aid of videos, books, or classes. Activated by some instinct, they approach the task without fear or inhibition, resolving to do no more than get up on their feet and see what happens. Setbacks do not deter them: when they fall, they get up and try again. Because they are totally relaxed, they do not hurt themselves. Adults on the sidelines fussing over minor bumps and bangs create inhibitions that can make the next task seem more of a hurdle.

MAKING PROGRESS

Like any part of the body that has not been exercised for some time, the mind will at first resist efforts to bring it under control. Instead of tackling unruly thoughts and feelings directly, yoga uses physical techniques to gain control of the mind. A difficult asana may take months to achieve. After trying and failing for weeks, a student may succeed in holding the boat pose for a wobbly second or two. Perseverance pays, and the pose can be held for a second longer every day. This is mind control in action.

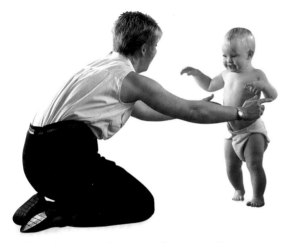

Children have the advantage of instinctual spontaneity as they approach physical challenges.

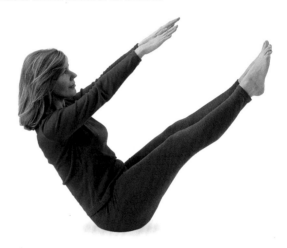

The boat posture demands perfect control of several major muscles.

EXERCISING THE MIND

A good way to begin the conscious practice of mind control is to choose a point in the week and sit quietly for five minutes with your eyes closed, listen to your breathing, let it slow down, and just feel at peace. Then increase the sessions to ten minutes, to three times a week, and then to once a day. Do this at about the same time every day, for discipline is an important aspect of mental control.

Sit erect but comfortable on your heels or in a cross-legged position on the floor. Raise your head so that your gaze is directly ahead, then close your eyes. Rest your hands palm upward on your knees with your thumb and fingertips touching.

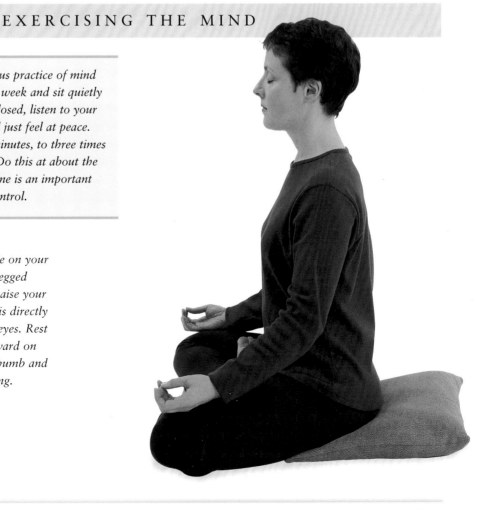

Visualization

································

The mind's eye is always on standby to access images from memory that will help the mind understand anything from instructions for finding a street in a strange city to a talk on politics. Yoga harnesses the mind's ability to visualize in order to overcome blockages. Imagining the hands reaching up to the sky during an upward stretch can induce the spine to stretch that little bit further. Recalling a wonderful day sunbathing on a tropical beach helps the muscles relax more deeply after stretching.

While the mind is trying to visualize what a person might look like from a description, its hidden eye is at work behind the scenes, building up a picture the mind can use from the memory's Identikit store. Using the mind's eye consciously to aid body function and movement requires practice, since at first, self-consciousness can inhibit the imagination.

The technique of visualization therefore needs to be treated as a routine part of practice, like the stretches and the asanas. The body needs to be erect, while comfortable and relaxed, for a visualization session, so a few minutes need to be spent breathing and eliminating tension. Visualization is, in fact, more the creation of mood than the recall of a visual image, so many people find it easiest to recapture their feelings from some occasion such as a festival or a vacation, when they felt wonderful. After just a few sessions,

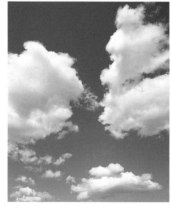

Visualizing a peaceful scene from nature can have a marked effect in calming the body.

visualization should become a habit, used regularly as a way of working at stretches and asanas, relaxing, overcoming stress, and lifting moods.

Imagination is a powerful and underused force. Writers on visualization always tell the story of a renowned 20th-century Indian yogi, Swami Rama, who took part in experiments at the Menninger Institute in the US. By visualizing a blue sky with small puffs of cloud floating almost motionless in it, he considerably slowed his heartbeat. In visualization, concentration persuades the brain that the image is reality, and the brain sends out signals to adjust the body's functions to what it perceives to be the mind's real state.

Interest in the healing power of visualization has increased in recent years. It has been found to be effective in alleviating asthma, and even in helping disabled people to regain some mobility. There is currently controversy over its role in causing remission in serious diseases, such as multiple sclerosis and cancer. Until more research has been done, the degree to which visualization can be effective in curing and preventing illness will not become clear. What is certain, however, is that, carried out regularly and properly, visualization can speed healing and alleviate suffering, reduce pain and lift the spirits, making illness easier to bear. The key to success is total concentration, and using the mind's eye is an important technique in meditation, which is the heart of yoga.

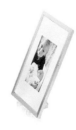

Visualize your hands reaching out to someone you love during a forward bend. You may find you can reach your toes.

PRACTICING VISUALIZATION

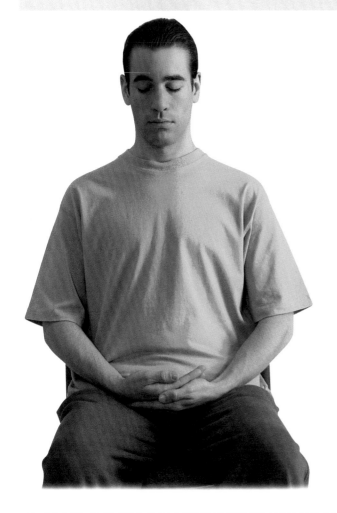

Choose a convenient time and a quiet place for your practice sessions, and spend some time before the first one deciding on the subject of your visualization. Sessions should last about 10 minutes at first, but as you gain confidence you will find that you can concentrate for longer and practice will last for up to 20 minutes.

1 Sit erect on a chair or on the floor and make yourself comfortable. Check that your head is balanced and your feet flat on the floor. Join your hands in your lap. Shrug your shoulders and check yourself from head to toe, contracting and releasing muscles to relieve any tension. Close your mouth and breathe steadily and rhythmically through your nose for several minutes, concentrating on the sound of your breathing and on feeling peaceful. When you feel relaxed, turn your mind gently to the subject of your visualization, focusing on the atmosphere and the associated mood rather than the visual scene.

2 Maintaining your breathing rhythm, dwell for a while in the inner world you have created, letting it surround you. As it begins to fade, try to retain the mood and feeling it brought. When the image has gone, open your eyes and stretch gently.

OVERCOMING INSOMNIA

Insomnia is a disorder experienced by almost everyone at some time. It can be relieved through visualization, which works by helping the mind and body calm down before sleeping. If your thoughts are racing, slow them by thinking of an image to visualize – a flower or a tranquil landscape you know and love at the close of the day.

3 As you move your fingers, imagine the tranquil beauty of a flower. Breathing slowly, focus on this peaceful scene until you feel suffused with its calm.

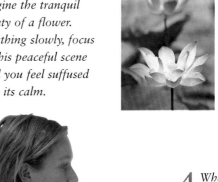

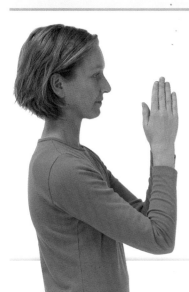

1 Raise your hands in front of your face with fingers and thumbs touching.

2 Breathe out, and open out your fingers and thumbs, imagining them to be the opening petals of a flower.

4 When you feel ready, imagine the light fading at the end of the day and the lily's petals closing tight. As you do so, close your fingers and prepare to sleep.

Meditation

....

The mind loves routine and thrives on expectation, so in a sense just heading for a quiet place at a preplanned time and sitting there for a few minutes, breathing quietly and calming the thoughts, counts as a meditation session. Like everything else, meditation takes time and has to begin somewhere.

There are, in fact, few rules governing meditation and everyone's objective should be to discover the way that suits them best. To begin with, it is sensible to make a routine of meditating in the same quiet place at the same time every week, or twice a week, or preferably every day. Immediately after a meal is not a good time, since digestion uses energy and causes sleepiness. Lying down also causes drowsiness, and standing can be a strain, so it is better to sit on the floor or in a chair.

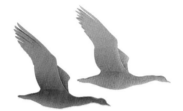

The wild goose is a traditonal focus for meditation.

First sessions should normally last for about ten minutes, and the first few minutes should be spent concentrating on breathing steadily and rhythmically, and encouraging a pleasant feeling of relaxation and peacefulness. The next stage is to focus the mind on a single thought. The difference between relaxation and meditation is that during meditation the mind remains aware of the body and its presence in place and time, but withdraws from the scene and focuses its energy on one, nonphysical object. At first, however, many people find it easier to visualize a physical image.

In the beginning it may be impossible to focus the mind for more than a few seconds before something intervenes or the image fades. It is important not to allow feelings of disappointment or failure to take over, but to continue concentrating on the sound and rhythm of your breathing. During the next session the image, which is now more strongly associated with a feeling of tranquility and the regular rhythm of the breath, may be recalled for longer. There will inevitably be days when, for a variety of reasons, recall and concentration will seem altogether impossible, but with regular practice control of the mind will gradually strengthen, so that the peaceful effect of the image will persist and deepen.

End each session by concentrating on the breathing as the image fades. The deeper the concentration, the more relaxed the body, so people who have been meditating do not feel stiff after they open their eyes and rarely need to stretch. Meditating leaves the mind feeling tranquil and positive, and the body comfortable.

POSTURE FOR MEDITATION

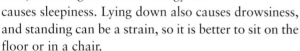

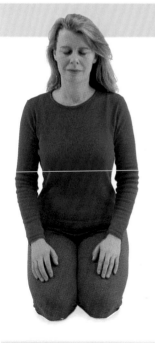

Left: *Discomfort destroys concentration, so you should wear unrestricting clothing and sit in a comfortable position. If you think it will be easier, meditate in a kneeling position, sitting back on your heels, but lift your trunk and head so that the body is balanced and never allow yourself to sink onto your hips.*

Right: *There are good physical reasons for the traditional cross-legged meditation positions: the erect posture facilitates effective breathing, which fuels the electromagnetic circuits between body and brain. Joining the hands in the lap completes an energy circuit – electrodes on the fingertips show that some ten millivolts leaks out. And closing the eyes shuts out distractions.*

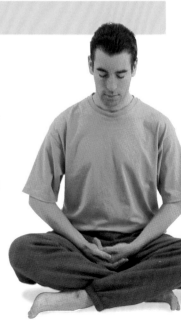

HALF-LOTUS AND LOTUS

HALF-LOTUS

When you are able to sit cross-legged for more than ten minutes without feeling any strain, you can try the half-lotus. It is important, however, not to try this position if your joints and muscles are not sufficiently flexible since there is a danger of damage from straining the groin.

Sit in a simple cross-legged position, with the right ankle crossing over the left. Check that your posture is erect. Push your left heel as far in toward your groin as you can. Now grasp your left ankle with both hands and lift your foot, placing it on your left thigh joint. The sole of your left foot should face upward.

LOTUS (PADMASANA)

Some people are so flexible they can sit in the lotus position without any difficulty at all. If you find it hard, however, you should not try to teach yourself to do it. It is best learned with a teacher who can assess your flexibility and help you to progress through the correct exercises.

THE MUDRAS

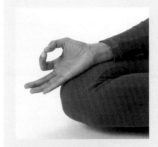

The Jnana mudra is traditionally used for meditation. Sit comfortably erect and bend your index fingers into your thumbs, then place your hands on your knees, palms upward.

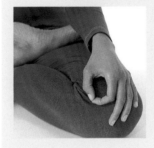

Bhoomi sparsh mudra is a pose in which the Buddha is often represented. With the tips of your thumbs and index fingers touching, rest the palms of your hands on your knees.

Half-lotus

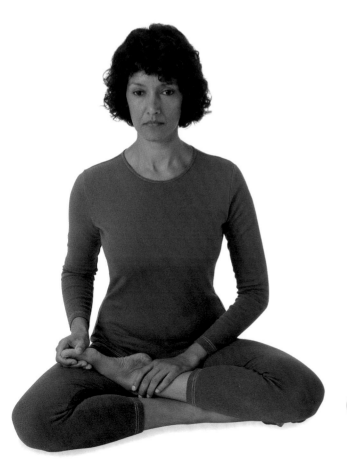

Lotus

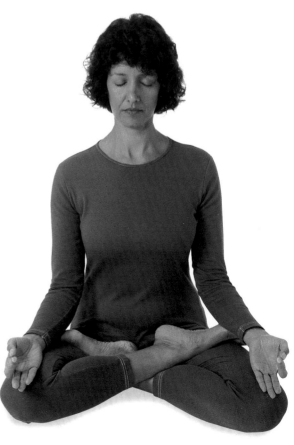

The Goal of Meditation

The elusive ability to concentrate is mastered by practicing meditation regularly and often. Gradually, the object or the image or sound on which the mind is focused fills the consciousness more completely, for longer. With practice, meditation, like anything else, becomes more natural. It becomes easier to relax on a crowded train at the end of a busy day by withdrawing and, while remaining aware of the surroundings, relaxing into a quieter existence for a few reviving moments. Later it becomes possible to withdraw into a meditative state without the aid of an external object, such as a candle or a mantra.

There are countless meditation systems and they attract different types of people. One of the objectives of yoga is to open the mind and make it more receptive, so it is essential not to remain too closely involved with one meditation school. Meditation should be progressive and a system that is not helpful at the start may become meaningful later on.

A need to relax, to calm down, is a good reason for meditating. It has a calming influence from the beginning, because just sitting for ten minutes, breathing quietly, and trying to focus the mind on something external has a tranquilizing effect. In a deeper sense, however, meditation is calming because it releases the consciousness from concern with the everyday difficulties that seem to paralyze it, freeing it to discover other realities. One may become aware that philosophical questions, such as the purpose of living or the nature of consciousness, are important. Such thoughts may persist for the briefest of moments, but they put the pettiness of everyday existence in perspective. An inner tranquility comes from understanding that we are part of more than our body and our life. And bothersome problems may be unexpectedly simple to solve after meditating.

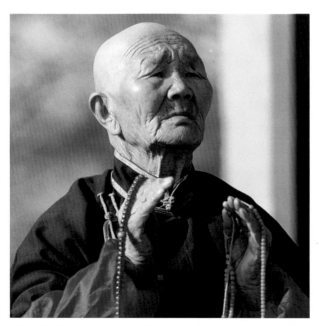

Mystical union with the divine is a feature of many belief systems, such as Christianity, Sufism, and Buddhism, and deep meditation is frequently the means of access to this visionary state. This picture shows a Buddhist priest meditating with the aid of beads.

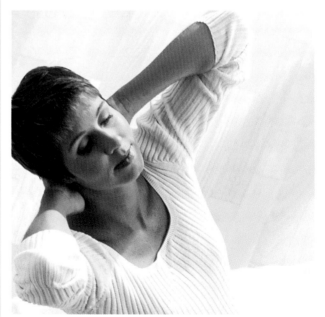

Withdrawing from the press of activity that usually surrounds us has many benefits. At a simple level it allows the mind to relax and become calm. At a deeper level it may perhaps give us a sense of a realm beyond our everyday existence.

Meditation elevates the mind, leaving the body to carry on without the influence of the consciousness. That is the meaning of one often-repeated statement: "I am not a body." Lifting the pressure seems to give the body a chance to run a fault-checking program over its essential circuits – its immune system and other vital processes – repair some of the damage caused by stress and ward off illness. Meditation can help clear up a cough or a cold.

Some people are naturally contemplative and find meditation playing a progressively more significant role in their lives. These personalities seem most fitted to follow the path of raja yoga, the ancient yoga of the mind, regarded by all who practice yoga as the most advanced school and the most fulfilling. Only a few people feel called to pursue raja yoga. It demands immense self-discipline and highly evolved powers of concentration. Its ideals are to discover the true Self beneath the image projected by the ego, and to experience reality undistorted by incomplete sensory impressions. The ultimate reward is the achievement of the mystical state of samadhi, or union with the cosmic self. There are no short cuts, and the attainment of samadhi is a task that will take the best part of a lifetime.

Asked to define the goal of meditation, most people would almost certainly expect the answer to be "to achieve enlightenment." On the contrary, however, meditation must have no goal. It is a voyage of exploration, which leads everyone along a different path. Approaching it with a goal in mind is to start out with the autopilot set on a destination. Meditation is the opposite of following a predetermined course, or even of searching. Samadhi comes only by surprise; the more one searches, the more elusive it is. The goal is to meditate and to enjoy the sense of wonder that is perhaps life's greatest reward.

A lighted candle can provide a focus for meditation.

AIDS TO CONCENTRATION

People are all different and some find it natural to meditate. People with strong religious beliefs have often been encouraged to meditate by repetition of the litany or other practices of their church. Many Christians find it natural to meditate on the words or image of Jesus Christ. Others may need to experiment with different devices before they find a few words, an image such as a lighted candle, an object such as a pebble, or perhaps a sound that strikes a chord within their mind. For thousands of years yogis have meditated to the sacred sound of Om (au-uu-m), which concentration will amplify until it fills body, mind, and the universe.

One classic Buddhist form of meditation is to count the breaths up to ten and back down again to one, and keep doing that until the mind is concentrating totally on the breathing. A heartfelt need to improve concentration is a common reason for meditating, and breathing is the first form

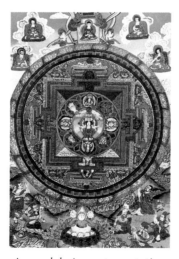

A mandala is a representation of the universe, usually in circular form, which is often used as a focus for meditation.

of concentration. Becoming absorbed in the breathing is a way of concentrating on life and the desire to live. Everyone desires to be absorbed in something – a movie, a hobby, another person. Meditation taken past the first stages satisfies this need totally. People from the Buddha to 20th-century yogis have spoken of being absorbed in a oneness with a universal consciousness.

At the beginning, when it may be hard to focus the mind, do not hesitate to try anything that helps you concentrate, be it a device like those illustrated here, a mental image or an inspiring text. Just as practice perfects the asanas, however, you will find your ability to focus your mind improves in time and you will then be able to meditate without the help of external aids to concentration.

An ancient "om" symbol, used as an aid to meditation.

Since ancient times beads have been used as an aid to prayer and meditation.

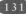

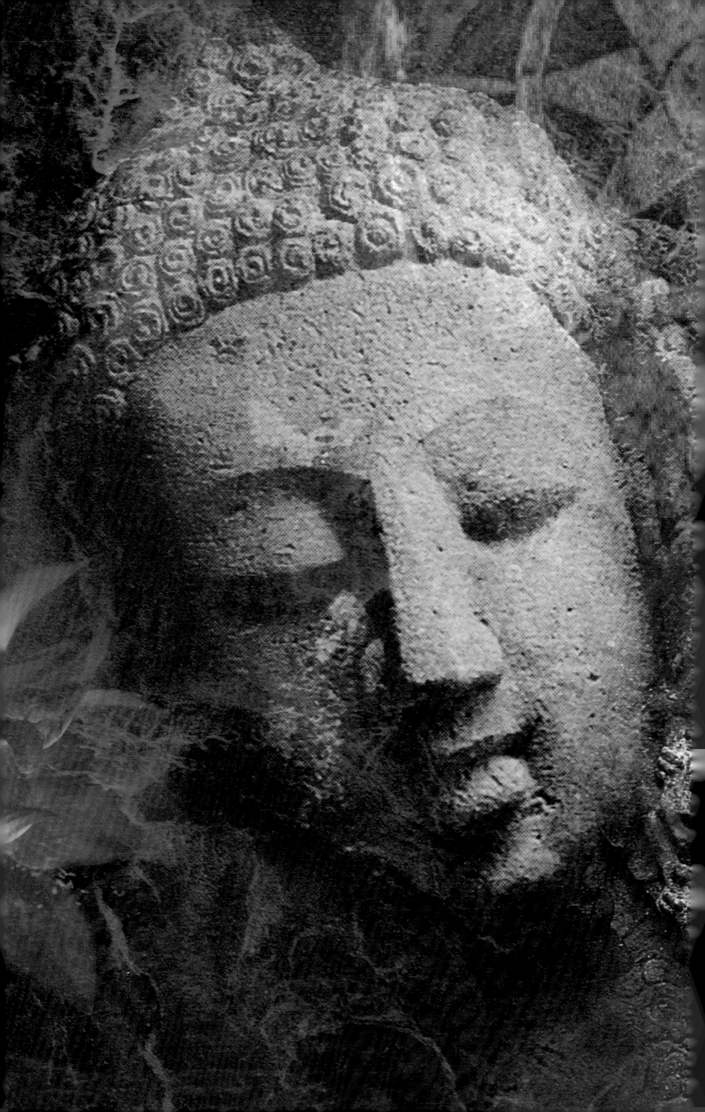

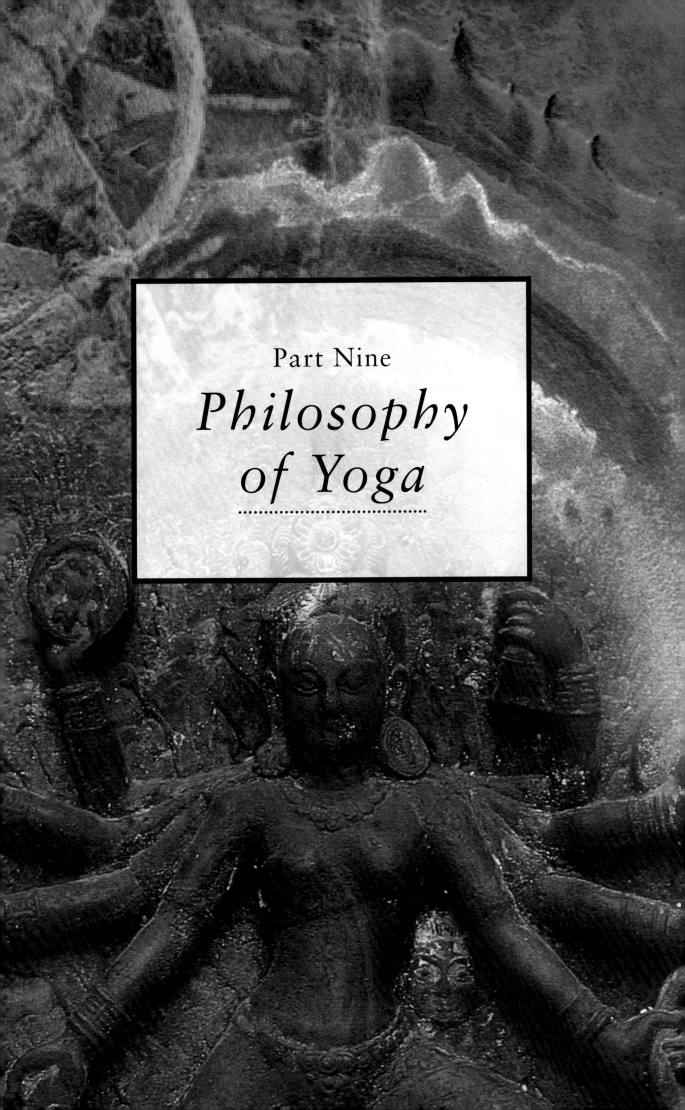

Part Nine

Philosophy
of Yoga

How We Treat Ourselves

Inner peace is the key to health and the goal of yoga.

Yoga not only involves practicing special techniques, it offers a unique approach to life. The classic texts, such as those of the sage Patañjali, offer a set of principles to govern the way we treat ourselves, called niyamas; and five yamas or restraints to be observed when dealing with other people. These niyamas and yamas correspond to the teachings of the principal religions – they read something like the ten commandments of Christianity – but they involve a different understanding of life.

More than two millennia ago the yoga sages worked out that what we call morality or ethics is not just a set of socially desirable rules, it is a practical necessity. Through meditation they had gained an early realization that, ultimately, life is an intricate pattern of energy fields. These days, yogis and many scientists are united in seeing existence in this way. The rhythms, sometimes called bodytime, of the energy fields governing the workings of the body and mind have a harmony, they believe, and if it is interrupted, physical and mental ill health result. Assuming that there is a natural tendency toward harmony, failure to observe the niyamas and yamas must set up harmful vibrations.

An electrocardiogram of a damaged heart reveals the harmful effects anger can have. Similarly, telling lies can produce psychophysical problems for the perpetrator. If, therefore, people behave antisocially, they damage the harmonious flow of their energy fields, and attempting yoga practice will add to the conflict. How can anyone who has just deceived a friend or injured someone in a fight concentrate their energies on meditation? Accordingly, the yoga sages realized that if people want a sense of internal peace they have to control the ways in which they act, first in regard to themselves and then to others.

In today's world, it is becoming increasingly difficult to achieve inner harmony. Yoga is one way to begin to rectify the harmful effects of modern life. The yamas and the niyamas together form one element in the complex philosophy of yoga, which has evolved over centuries to give guidance to people on how to achieve harmony of the body and peace of mind. The following pages describe some of its many branches, from shauca, (achieving inner and outer purity) to santosha (learning to accept situations in life with equanimity) and explain how to apply their principles and guidelines to the demands of modern life.

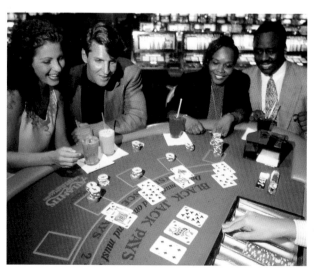

A visit to a casino seems pleasant to some, but others see it as enslavement to false objects of desire.

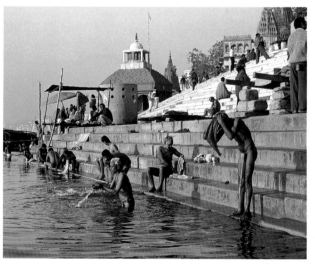

Spiritual and bodily cleanliness have always been important in India, where yoga originated.

THE FIVE NIYAMAS

ONE
To maintain a state of mental purity and physical cleanliness

The niyamas begin with shauca, which means inner and outer purity. Inner purity is regarded as purity of mind, and this, says Vyasa, "should be known to arise from righteousness and spiritual knowledge." Great importance has always been attached to outer cleanliness. Even today, Indians forced to live on the streets frequently wash at standpipes. Seldom is a really unclean person to be seen, no matter how poor they are.

TWO
To rise above objects of desire

Yoga enjoins its followers to practice austerity, but in moderation: not to eat too little, nor too much; not to sleep too little, nor too much. This form of austerity, called tapas, leans more toward the balanced control of the senses than the asceticism of some religious orders. It translates as seeing clearly how to modify action so that we limit the punishment we give ourselves from indulging in excesses, and so allow body and mind to operate to their fullest capacity.

THREE
To accept our situation in life with equanimity

Santosha – equanimity – recognizes that where we are now in life is definitive: this is the point to which we have brought ourselves. We will be happiest if we accept it without regret or resentment, which are a major cause of illness. Recognizing that we can only start out from the position we are in now helps us maintain a calm, dispassionate attitude, even when our lives are in a state of crisis.

FOUR
To repeat sacred words

Only by reading can we discover the spiritual thoughts of great people of the past or the present which speak to us. A few minutes a day spent reading ancient texts and scriptures, philosophy, or poetry reminds us to continue working toward something better, more fulfilling than the world of pressures, manipulation, and artificiality that surrounds us now.

FIVE
To be devoted to God – the life force

We must accept that we can never completely understand the miracle of the universe, and so we must surrender to God, if we have religious beliefs, or, if we are not religious, to wonder – and a sense of joy at being part of such wonder.

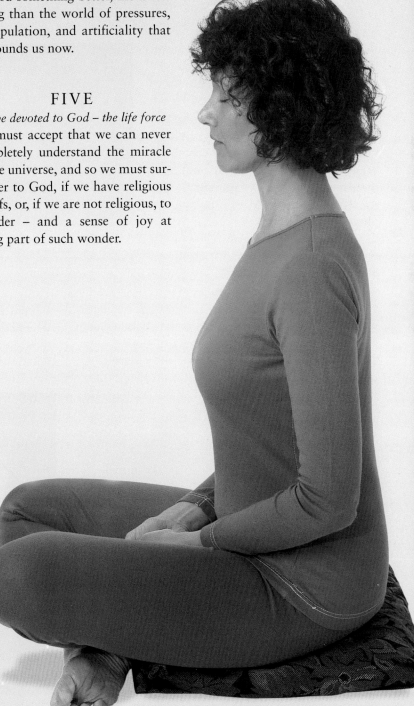

Dealing with Other People

The great spiritual teachings have much in common, most notably their rules of behavior. All have urged us to treat others as we would have them treat us. These similarities come as no surprise to followers of yoga, who believe that the universe and its inhabitants are subject to a network of laws governing thought and action. People may choose whether to obey them, but if they do not, they will not feel happy and may not remain healthy.

Almost everyone can remember disregarding the rule, "Do as you would be done by," with disastrous effects on peace of mind. And by revealing instances of how the interplay between thoughts and body affects energy and health, modern research supports the idea that illness can result from mental and physical disharmony.

The classic yoga sages set out the yamas as guidelines for our behavior toward other people. There are five principal yamas, but some texts list up to ten. Some may be read as examples, rather than taken literally. Ksama, for instance, exhorts everyone to accept abuse or apparent ill treatment quietly and not to respond in kind, like Christ turning the other cheek. It may be interpreted in a modern sense as good advice on refusing to let people irritate you.

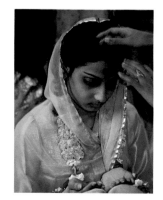

Faithfulness in sexual relationships is one aspect of right living.

Failing to obey these 2,000-year-old principles will, even now, do nobody any good. The injunction not to get involved in violence, for example, stems from understanding that thought vibrations that cause violent action only result in more violence, harming the attacker and the victim. In yoga, the end never justifies violent means, even if the goal is to overthrow a tyrant.

Yoga does not only set rules, it provides workable techniques for training oneself to follow them. It teaches mind and body how to calm ruffled emotions and stifle society's conditioning to reply in kind, so that the senses remain under the will's command in all circumstances. Medical research into stress during the 20th century has demonstrated the effectiveness of the yoga approach.

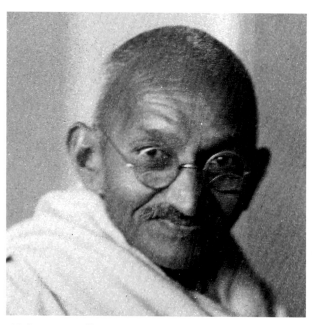

Mahatma Gandhi inspired millions with his refusal to use violence in his struggle for Indian independence.

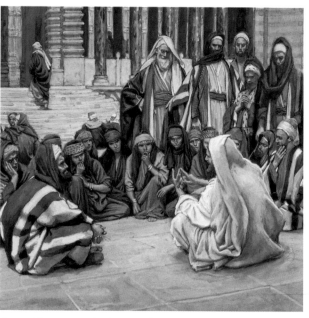

Jesus Christ preached nonviolence as a way of life, turning the other cheek as the answer to hostility.

THE FIVE YAMAS

ONE

To refrain from violence, in thought, word, or deed

The elimination of all violence from our relationships with others is the first yama, called ahimsa. This means never blaming other people for things that happen; never speaking harsh words to another; never hurting any person by thought, speech, or action; and never killing anyone. Since World War II it has become almost acceptable for a head of state to take military action to prevent worse violence by an enemy state. Yet the principle of ahimsa was the one adopted by Mahatma Gandhi when he urged that perceived wrongs should never be opposed by the further wrong of violence.

TWO

To refrain from stealing

Asteya means never taking anything that belongs to others. It extends beyond the theft of objects to include possessions in the widest sense. Wrongfully appropriating thoughts and ideas is theft, too. In modern society a lot of stealing goes on under the guise of being alert and competitive in a hard commercial world.

THREE

To avoid covetousness

Yoga teachings do not demand a vow of poverty, but they insist that possessiveness should be avoided. True peace of mind does not come from collecting material objects. If we make a point of holding on to them we create harmful inhibitions in ourselves and in those with whom we are in contact.

FOUR

To speak the truth

The sage Vyasa defined truth as follows: "that which is beneficial to beings, spoken justly, and the agreeable is also said to be true." In other words, there is a tendency for us to tell half-truths in order to save ourselves embarrassment – or to gain some benefit or even to wound. Satya means always speaking the truth. In the end it will bring the greatest benefit.

FIVE

To refrain from sexual depravity

The yamas were once generally expounded to members of religious groups, who had taken vows to remain celibate. For others, brahmacharya may be interpreted as "love, not lust, and faithfulness in marriage." Strict social rules governing normal sexual behavior may not be as relevant as they once were, yet this yama is still necessary. The effects of the actions of those who give way to depraved lust cause indescribable misery to children forced into prostitution in countries all over the world.

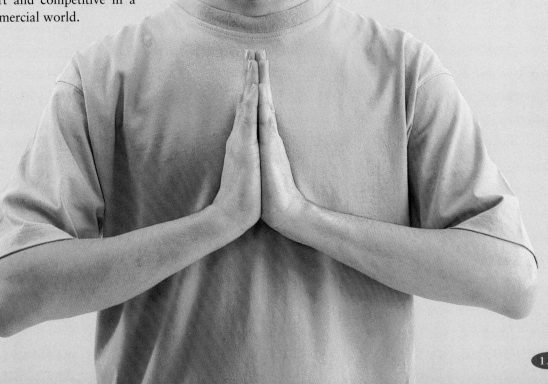

Karma Yoga

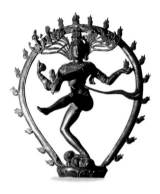

Shiva, Hindu god of good and evil, creation and destruction, dancing.

Karma yoga is the yoga of selfless action. This concept was first expounded in the Bhagavad Gita, *which, through its descriptions of the rivalries of two great clan families, speaks of spiritual duty. The* Bhagavad Gita *was written by the sage Vyasa, who is thought to have lived sometime between 500 and 200* BCE. *It may have been written as the Hindu answer to the challenge of Buddhism, which arose in India around 500* BCE.

At that time, karma yoga was a revolutionary new yoga. Instead of being concerned only with meditation and asceticism, like jnana yoga, or the worship of a supreme being, like bhakti yoga, it is concerned with ordinary, everyday living.

One of the most important things the *Bhagavad Gita* did was give yoga (which at the time was based almost exclusively on experience during meditation) an official philosophy that linked it both to the concepts of the universe set out in the ancient scriptures,

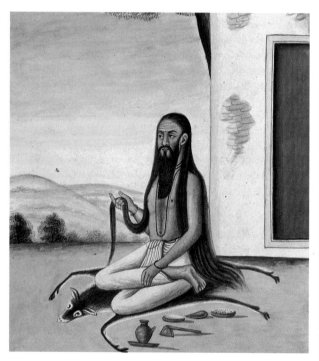

A yogi is one who is not anxious about the future, Krishna tells Arjuna in the Bhagavad Gita. The yogi, he says, should find a solitary place and live alone there. All his time should be spent sitting with an erect spine and the eyes focused on the end of the nose, keeping perfectly still and meditating on the Self.

and the new beliefs emerging at that time. It speaks, for instance, of the ancient concept of Brahman at the center of the universe, the still, small voice within the Self that may be heard through meditation. And it elaborates on the doctrine of karma, an idea common to the emerging Jain and Buddhist religions.

Karma is a Sanskrit word meaning action or work. The doctrine of karma is that everyone's present circumstances are the result of actions in the past – and, of course, that future actions will affect what happens to them in the future. This doctrine has a connection with the idea of reincarnation: that actions in this life can determine one's destiny after death, in future incarnations. However, karma is an impersonal law of cause and effect, entirely separate from belief in a supreme being who punishes or forgives wrongdoing.

When people hear about karma yoga they often think it is about doing good works, helping with the chores, and giving money to charity, in order to gain spiritual credits. Its meaning is much wider, however. It is about the whole process of action in life. As human beings we cannot avoid acting. Even if all we do is sit and breathe, that will soon start having consequences. Yoga understands that every day we deal with the effects of previous causes, and that the actions we take to deal with them create new effects.

The outcome of every daily disappointment is affected by the way it is handled when it arises – and the outcome of even minor annoyances can affect one's mood and outlook. Moreover, the consequences of past actions can interfere with one's ability to deal satisfactorily with other setbacks that may follow – as karma yoga teaches. Practiced regularly, yoga trains the mind to respond to all events with a peaceful, balanced attitude, based on the understanding that in the long term happiness and unhappiness balance out. "A yogi," the god Krishna tells Arjuna in the *Bhagavad*

Gita, "is one who is not anxious about the future." Eventually, with time and mental effort, the unflurried outlook that suffuses the mind and body after yoga becomes part of daily life. Until then, students have to visualize the goal at all times, training themselves to remain dispassionate so they can deal equably with all life's stresses, from the difficulties of meeting schedules to the problems of dealing with uncooperative families and noisy neighbours.

Karma yoga teaches that the best way to avoid creating detrimental effects is always to act in the most responsible way. It is important to see the situation and the consequences of possible actions clearly, and to take the correct action under the circumstances. It warns against acting with personal benefit in mind, to the extent of never doing something wrong, even if it is popular. Everyone's experience shows that well-intentioned actions often turn out wrong, but karma yoga answers that selfless decisions are most likely to have good consequences. Whatever the apparent outcome of any action, it is therefore important to remain dispassionate about it.

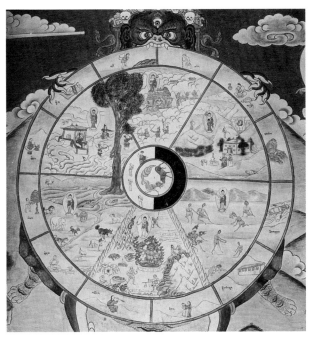

The Wheel of Life symbolizes the idea that with each action we take we release old karma and fill ourselves with new karma.

THE BHAGAVAD GITA

The Bhagavad Gita tells the story of a confrontation between two clans, the Kauravas and the Pandavas. Prince Arjuna, leader of the Pandavas, faces an agonizing moral dilemma as the battle lines are drawn up: it is his duty to order the battle to begin, but if he does he will be responsible for the deaths of members of his clan. He expresses his anguish to his charioteer, who reveals himself as the god Krishna, an incarnation of the gods Brahma, the creator, Siva the destroyer, and Vishnu the preserver. The epic consists of a spirited discussion of the duties of life between Arjuna and Krishna.

Arjuna belongs to the warrior caste, Krishna counsels, so it is his duty to fight. But the act of ordering the fighting to begin will, in the end, have been an effective decision. Action is unavoidable in life. Decisions must be taken on the basis of duty and not from selfish motives; having made a choice one must not worry about its results. This is karma yoga, which concerns itself only with what is happening in the present.

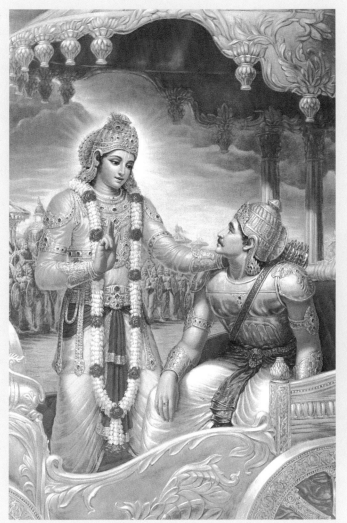

The god Krishna in the guise of a charioteer counsels the warrior-leader Arjuna on right action in the Bhagavad Gita.

The Spiritual Journey

Yoga is not something to be dabbled in. Working on the asanas alone and ignoring the meditative aspects is just touching the fringe. To begin yoga is to start on a spiritual journey which will lead to great self-awareness and fulfillment.

In essence, yoga trains the mind to approach life with equanimity, based on the understanding that in the long term, happiness and unhappiness balance out. This is the teaching of karma yoga, described on the preceding pages. Although this central philosophy of yoga can take years to understand, the benefits of the change in thinking it engenders become obvious in surprisingly practical ways very early on. Students end their yoga sessions bathed in tranquility and with a heightened awareness that helps them deal more successfully with everyday situations.

Yoga also teaches compassion and integration with others. But it believes that people should have true compassion, not superficial sympathy. Feeling sorry for someone who is ill, out of work, or living on the street is of no help to them. What they need is understanding, communication, and sharing in the form of practical help based on insight and given with no thought of a return. Yoga is not psychotherapy but

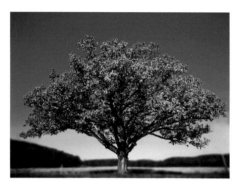

A tree, reaching from earth to heaven, changing with the seasons and so enduring for thousands of years, is a powerful symbol of hope and renewal.

it does encourage a realistic awareness of one's own shortcomings and a more understanding approach to other people. Yoga is a healing force which guides the personality toward integration of body and mind.

The need for this integration seems to have been growing steadily through the second half of the 20th century. The celebrated yogi Indra Devi wrote in 1998 – her 99th year – of the million people currently in psychiatric treatment in the USA, the million people there in the grip of alcohol abuse, the million and a half criminal offences committed each year, and the 20,000 suicides carried out successfully each year. While the broad view of meditation among people who do not practice it is that its purpose is to achieve a happy kind of mystic state of mind, Indra Devi stresses a more practical benefit. Increasing self-awareness is one of yoga's principal goals. Only through deeper self-knowledge will people find relief from tension, fear, anxiety, and boredom.

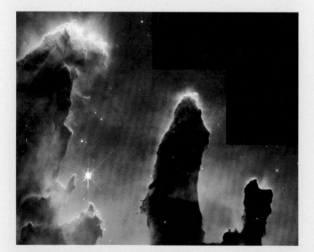

This image from the Hubble Space Telescope shows the formation of stars at the Eagle Nebula M16, also called "the hand of God."

THE YOGA OF DEVOTION

Yoga is a quest for spiritual enlightenment, not a religion, but it does not exclude religious belief. Bhakti is a Sanskrit word meaning "loving devotion to God leading to samadhi" and bhakti yoga is the yoga of devotion. Followers of bhakti yoga try to transcend the anchoring effect of the ego by devoted service to God. They seek their own personal way of serving God, some through religious devotion and others through service to other people. The way of bhakti yoga accords with the teachings of the world's great religions that through selflessly loving and serving others one can shake off the shackles of ego and truly love ourselves. The ideal of this classic school of yoga is to discover the true Self and through it, achieve unity with God.

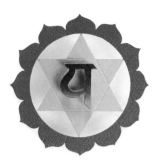

Energy becomes more spiritual as it rises from the base of the spine through the chakras to the head.

The integration of one's personality by means of self-awareness, and teaching oneself through exercise, relaxation, and breathing to control body and mind are the first stages of the spiritual journey yoga offers. One result of working toward integration is that you live life to the full, so yoga changes your perception of reality. Once that point is reached, yoga directs the awareness outward toward a more fulfilling communication with other people and a deeper understanding.

Every mind is unique, and karma yoga is one of a whole hierarchy of yogas, each of which offers a different spiritual path. Bhakti yoga draws the mind along the ancient way of devotion to a personal god, and of mysticism. Jnana yoga seeks to develop intuitive knowledge. And ultimately, all paths lead to the king of yoga, raja yoga, in which the individual seeks, through deep meditation, to free the mind into a state of spiritual unity with the universe.

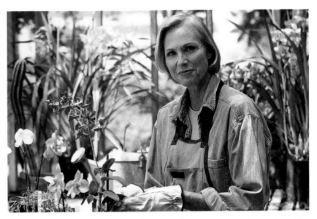

Yoga is any activity that brings about integration of body and mind, so there can be a yoga of dance, a yoga of music – even a yoga of gardening.

People who are half-hearted about yoga may still glimpse the benefits it can bring, but for them, practice does not lead to a happier life, just to a fractionally better one. If they then become discouraged and give up yoga, they are likely to remain more dissatisfied than if they had never glimpsed its rewards. In *The Yoga Sutras*, Patañjali comments that those who put in a little effort will benefit a little; while those who put in all their effort will reap the full physical and spiritual rewards.

EXPERIENCING TRANQUILITY

The mind can only be quiet when it is free from tension – yet tension often worsens if we complain about it or resist it. Inertia, expressed as a quiet submission, the capacity to accept things as they come, is the best tool to use to eliminate it. All yoga techniques – from poses to breath-retention to deep meditation – are directed toward helping people to cultivate a permanent sense of outward inertia and inner stillness. This enables us to face our tasks and the demands of daily life easily and calmly.

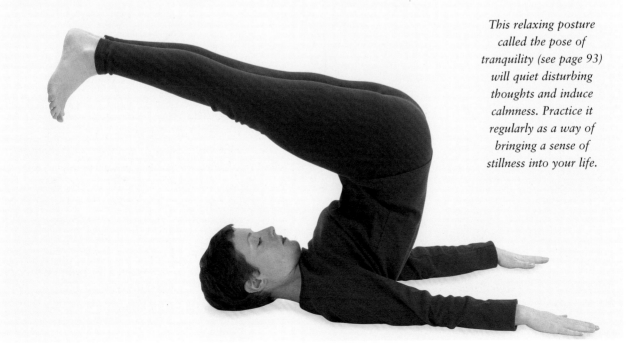

This relaxing posture called the pose of tranquility (see page 93) will quiet disturbing thoughts and induce calmness. Practice it regularly as a way of bringing a sense of stillness into your life.

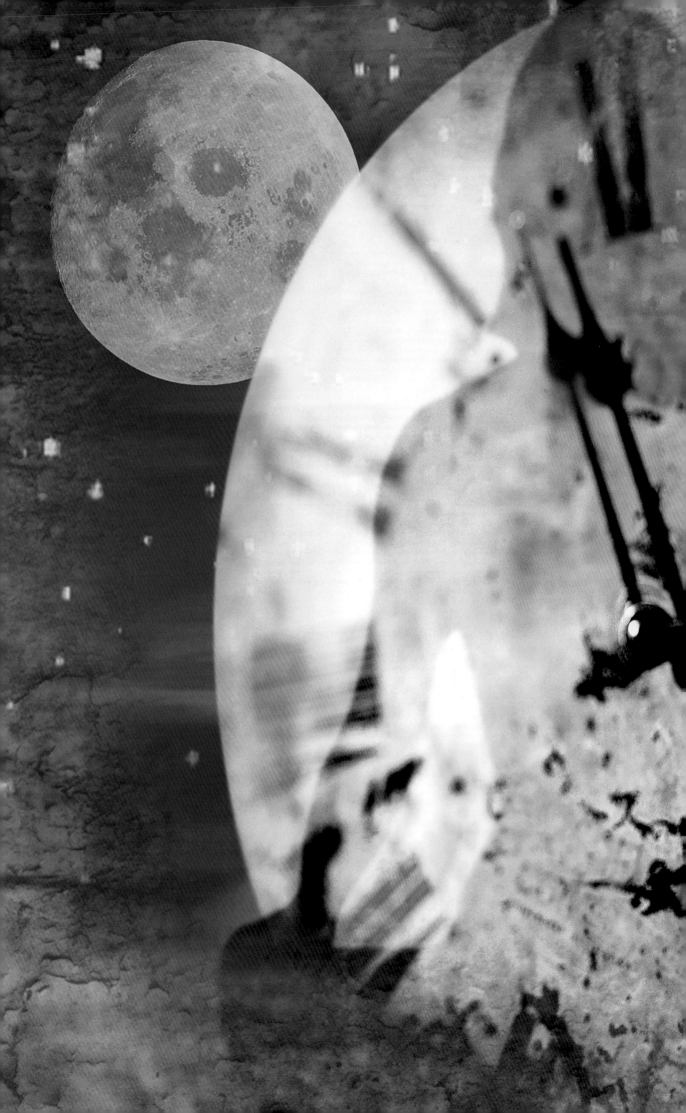

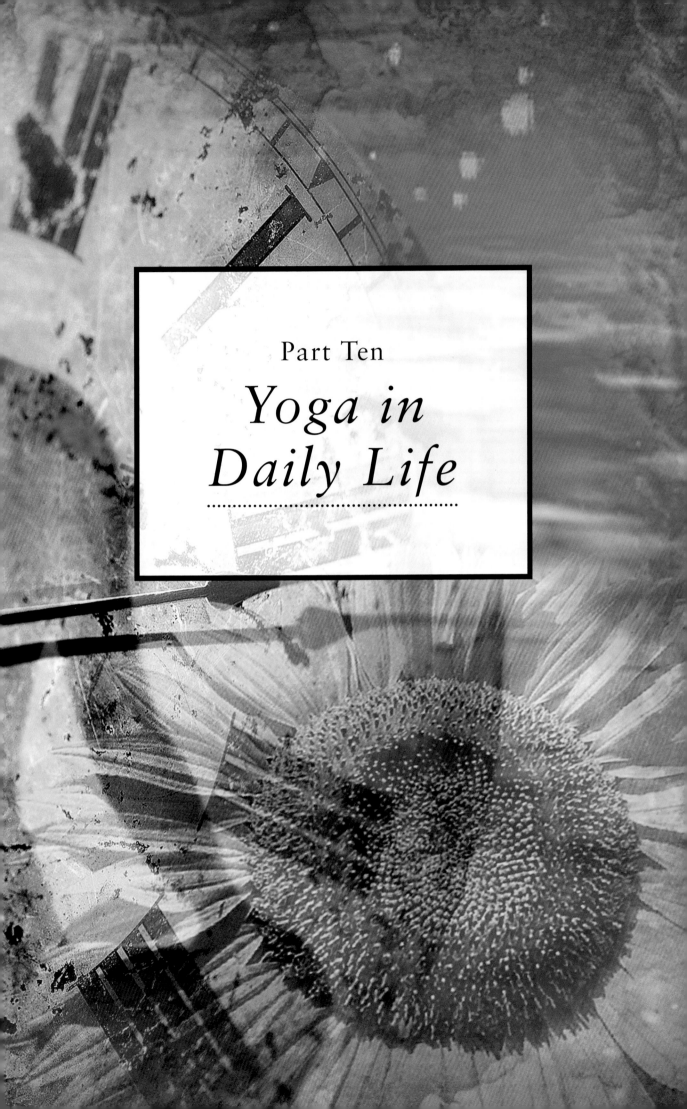

Part Ten

Yoga in Daily Life

Everyday Awareness

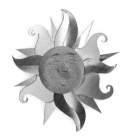

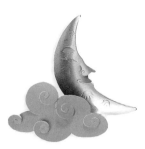

Because yoga is fundamentally holistic, its sages naturally pondered about what appear to be two separate aspects of existence: the physical and the spiritual. In yoga, the physical is called prakriti, or universal matter, and the spiritual purusha, or universal consciousness. The sages perceived prakriti and purusha as two forces, and existence as the interplay between them.

Three more forces link with this interplay. They are called gunas – the Sanskrit word for threads – and it is the intertwining of these threads that produces life. The pure life force, the first of these three threads, is called sattva; the second thread is the force of energy, called rajas; and tamas, the third thread, is the force of inertia. All three forces are present in every aspect of life.

The art of yoga is to establish the correct balance between the three gunas, and that affects the way the asanas, movements such as the bandhas, breathing, and the other yoga techniques are practiced. Although the theory outlined above may seem obscure and rather irrelevant to what takes place in a yoga class, when applied, it makes perfect sense. When practicing asanas, the principle of counterbalance is an effective way of ensuring that the body is not harmed by too much repetition of one exercise. For example, always following a backward bend with a forward bend improves the body's flexibility in all directions; always bending the spine in one direction is liable to damage it. However, since every aspect of yoga is holistic, the asanas do more than stimulate body systems, they also help free the life force or sattva, and establish a perfect balance between rajas and tamas.

One function of the asanas is to free the flow of prana, the life force.

This principle of balance applied to the mind explains why yoga tries to discourage the competitive spirit, in the sense of trying to outdo others instead of simply doing the best you can. Expressed theoretically, putting others down instead of strengthening oneself internally results in an imbalance of rajasic force. Yoga encourages sharing and participation instead of infighting and self-aggrandizement, an idea that has become a business theory during the 1990s, and is now taught in management schools.

The gunas have a relevance to every aspect of daily life. The following pages examine some of the ways in which they can be applied in order to bring harmony into everyday life.

THE SPIRIT OF FAIR PLAY

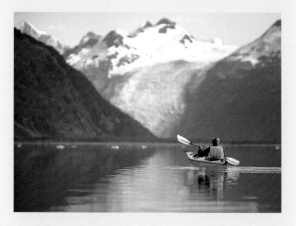

Yoga discourages cutthroat competition in any aspect of life, which it sees as unbalanced. One practical application of this idea is the use of relaxation and meditation as a way of improving performance at sports. Peak performance comes from achieving a high level of concentration and focusing the entire mind on doing the best you can do for your own fulfillment.

THE GUNAS

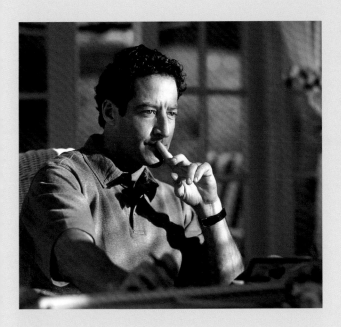

RAJAS
Type A people are rajasic types. They are deadline-conscious, competitive go-getters who knock others out along the way. They may have a great time for a while, but a rajasic way of life is unhealthy. Medical science has recently shown that these people are susceptible to stress-related diseases, such as heart attacks. In yogic theory, this is seen as the result of an excess of the rajasic force.

TAMAS
These types can broadly be distinguished as those exhibiting the "gasp syndrome" and those showing the "sigh syndrome." When something goes wrong with the gaspers, they tend to tense up under the strain, stick their chests out, and gasp with anger. The sighers do the opposite, they go limp, let their shoulders sag, and say "Oh no!" The name comes from the sign of hopelessness they always make. Tamas types are victims of lethargy and inertia. They tend to suffer from depression and illnesses associated with lack of energy, such as colds and ME.

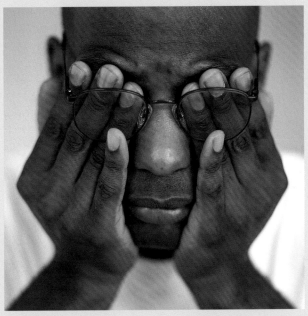

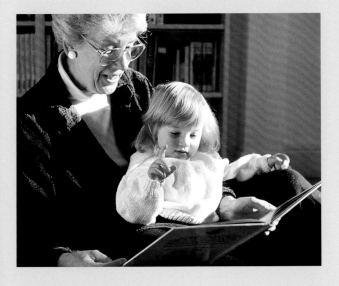

SATTVAS
Sattvas are the ones who strike a balance, the Type Bs, the compromisers and empathizers, those who are content to forego recognition if their actions will achieve some good. They are happy and healthy and they deal with problems dispassionately. Few people are naturally sattvic. Most of us fall here and there into the rajasic or tamasic camp, often in the way we tend to react to difficulties. Achieving a balanced personality is hard work and can take a lifetime to achieve.

Facing Problems

Yoga is a subtle yet powerful force for changing the personality. But unlike psychotherapy, it achieves this by looking to the present and the future, not by relying on finding the sources of all problems in the past. "Do the right thing, do it properly, and the right result will follow."

If the decision behind an action is wrong, the action will have bad consequences. What is needed is a clear view of the situation so that wise decisions may be taken and the best possible effects produced. Trying to explain a wrong action in terms of what happened in the past is a worthless exercise. The unconscious contains huge deposits of experience and memory, making it difficult to be sure that what psychotherapy uncovers is the root of the problem.

Yoga does not ignore the psychological past, but seeks to prevent psychotherapy becoming a crutch. It recognizes the essential role of therapy when, for example, a past trauma genuinely causes present problems. A multiple sclerosis patient, who complained of always feeling weak when she recalled the day her illness was diagnosed, became stronger after examining her shock with professional help. People who suffer trauma after a crash may have to recall the terrifying events so they may be released from the horror. The healing effects of psychotherapy counter the damage being wrought by the senses and allow the

mind to regain control. But psychotherapy is valueless when it is used to find excuses for wrong actions and bad decisions.

Everything in yoga helps to direct the thoughts toward the best way to act. It works to quieten the mind and bring it under control, leaving its owner free to contemplate alternatives instead of being carried along on a wave of emotion. Because yoga strengthens self-discipline, it also firms resolve, so that a decision to act is more likely to be carried out.

The three gunas present a model of the personality against which individuals can examine their reactions. Becoming aware of a tendency to respond with rajasic irritability to everyday events can start people working out ways of calming themselves. Anyone who feels they are only half living their life might consider trying to control the tamasic aspects of their personality. Few of us fail to derive a perverse satisfaction from things going wrong. Something makes us enjoy impressing people with the difficult times we are having, and believing that our sufferings are not understood.

THE BODY'S RESPONSE TO CHANGE

BLOOD PRESSURE RISES

HEART RATE INCREASES

BREATHING BECOMES ERRATIC

MUSCLES TENSE UP

When the mind is not at ease, the muscles tense up, the heart rate increases, the blood pressure rises. When danger threatens, these physical responses are essential lifesaving measures. But when they are the response to events that are not really threatening, they prevent the mind from making clear and rational responses, and they sap the body's natural energy flow. Everyday awareness means recognizing stressful situations as they arise and responding quickly by controlling the breathing, and by relaxing muscles that seem about to tense – the abdominal muscles, the muscles of the jaw, the mouth, and around the eyes. Concentrating on that for the few seconds it takes to relax disassociates the mind from the problem for long enough to be able to adopt a more detached and dispassionate attitude.

TAKING THE STRAIN

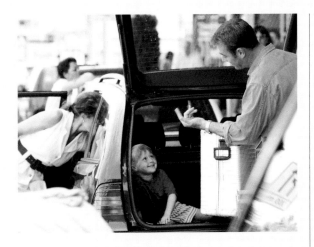

Car won't start? Caught in traffic? Missed the train? Kids late for school?

Do not allow start-of-the-day mishaps to raise your blood pressure. All these situations give you time to stop. Close your eyes, breathe for half a minute. Release your abdomen. Shrug your shoulders. Unclench your jaw. Close your eyes. Talk to your kids. Have a laugh. Then act. Use the time you have to spend waiting for the mechanic, a cab, or the next train to solve the problem, so the same thing does not happen again tomorrow.

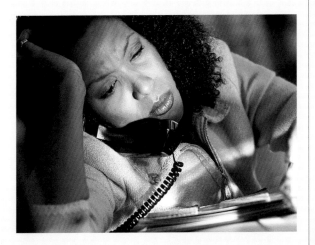

Having a bad time at work?

Take 5 minutes or more. Go somewhere you can be alone: a meeting room; the back stairs; the washroom; a public plaza at lunchtime. Sit down and close your eyes. Decide to work out how to deal with the problem after your break. Check your posture and give yourself five minutes of regular, satisfying, rhythmic breathing time to cool off. Visualize a tranquil scene that makes you feel peaceful and happy. The rest of the day might improve.

Screaming baby?

When a baby is screaming and you cannot see why, it is natural to panic. Lay the baby in a safe place and STOP. Go into another room, or just sit down. Close your eyes. Straighten your spine and lift your head. If necessary put your thumbs in your ears to block out the sound. Breathe calmly, deliberately, and rhythmically until you have relaxed and the feeling of panic has passed. Your state of calm will help both you and the baby.

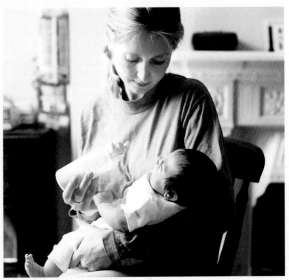

Road rage?

You are under threat from another driver, but if you are not in immediate danger you need not respond immediately. Gently straighten your spine, lower your shoulders, check that your head is balanced and relax your facial muscles. Breathe gently in and out a few times. Work out how to respond. Meet anger with calm and you will have a good chance of diffusing it.

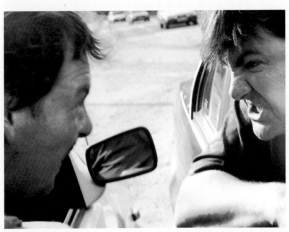

Controlling the Senses

In their true role, the senses are information gatherers at the service of the brain, whose transmissions enable us to decide how to act. But there is some tendency in the human psyche which drives us to gratify the senses addictively, so that their simple messages become monstrous demands.

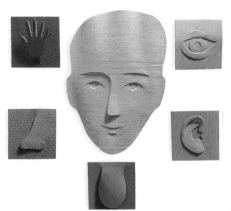

Yoga works in many ways to counteract this tendency. It emphasizes control, not only of the body but also of the mind, and especially of the senses.

Everyone has understood at some point how domineering the senses can become: the person who decides to cut down on chocolate, then starts bingeing; people just beginning their umpteenth attempt to give up smoking; or someone spending another day resentfully indoors because it is too cold to go out. Common experiences like these make the idea of controlling the senses seem improbable. Yet people who have lost the use of one of the senses offer proof of how dispensable they can be.

Yoga has gentle ways of teaching people how to control their senses. First, it relieves the tension resulting from being dominated by them. People sometimes take up yoga because they want to control their eating habits or weight problems. People with these preoccupations are often in a state of anxiety, and yoga teachers first encourage them to relax through stretching, breathing, and deep relaxation techniques. Yoga respects the body's natural design, and perceives that

metabolism has a role in its tendency to be slight or heavy. So apart from ensuring that the metabolism is stimulated through appropriate asanas, teachers will ignore the perceived weight problem. However, since yoga helps develop the ability to control the mind, students who persist with their practice will, in time, find that they are able to control the amount of food they eat.

Simply having the self-discipline to practice yoga techniques regularly and often, and to improve concentration, visualization, and meditation, teaches self-control. It is astonishing how powerful these techniques can be. What once brought yoga to the amazed attention of the sceptical Western world was the ability of famous yogis to demonstrate spectacular feats, such as raising their body temperature while standing half-naked for prolonged periods in subzero temperatures, or lying on beds of nails yet somehow appearing to feel no pain. Their mastery of the senses comes from practicing the basic yoga techniques with dedication and complete belief in their efficacy, and improving them over many years.

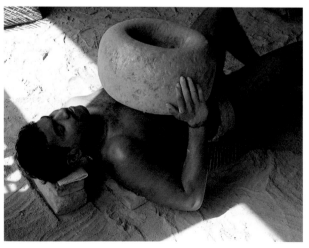

An Indian yogi demonstrates mastery of the senses by lying on a bed of nails supporting a heavy stone.

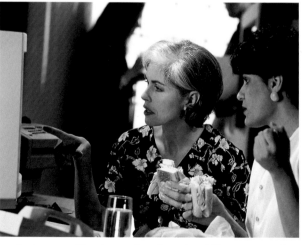

Instant gratification undermines the ability to control eating habits, resulting in illness.

OVERCOMING THE HEAT

The Sanskrit name for this asana is sitkari. This word sit means "cold" – this asana cools the body and relieves thirst. If you have high blood pressure, do it without holding your breath.

1 *Sit cross-legged on the floor, or stand with your feet a little apart, erect but relaxed. Breathe out. Purse your lips and fold the edges of your tongue upward to form a narrow channel.*

2 *Inhale slowly and deeply, sucking the air in through the channel in your tongue. Withdraw your tongue into your mouth, close your eyes, and hold your breath for up to half a minute, then breath out slowly and evenly through both nostrils.*

3 *Repeat steps 1 and 2 four or five times, concentrating on the pleasantly cooling sensation of the air passing over your tongue.*

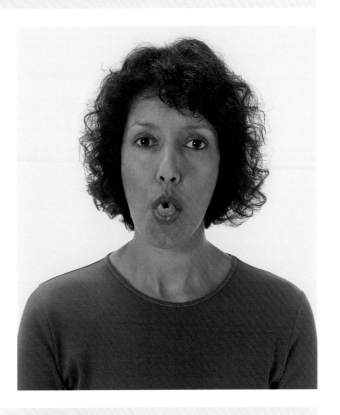

OVERCOMING THE COLD

Deep concentration persuades the brain to accept the mind's impression instead of the body's sensation. Speeding the blood circulation with these two simple exercises will give you a sense of warmth if you feel cold. While you are doing them, tell yourself how warm you feel instead of thinking about how cold you are.

1 *Sit on your heels with your spine erect and breathe rhythmically for a few minutes. Lay your arms on your thighs, and make fists with your hands. Breathe in and, holding your breath, bend forward slowly until your forehead touches your fists. Hold the position, breathing slowly in and out, for as long as you feel comfortable. Slowly straighten up, breathing in.*

2 *Stand erect with your hands by your sides and breathe rhythmically for a minute or two. On an out-breath, close your left nostril with the third finger of your right hand, and breathe in deeply through your right nostril. Now replace your right arm by your side, hold your breath, and tense every muscle from head to toe as hard as you can until your body begins to shudder. Breathe out slowly through both nostrils and relax.*

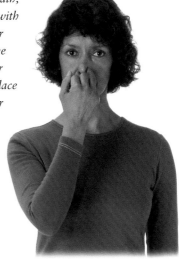

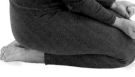

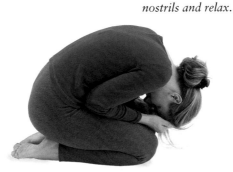

CAUTION

If you suffer from a heart condition, high blood pressure, or chest problems do not attempt these postures.

Yoga and Communication

Many people imagine students in yoga classes as groups of isolated individuals silently struggling to twist their bodies into unreal positions. In real yoga classes teacher and students talk while they stretch and twist. It helps them relax and can make difficult postures easier to achieve. Yoga aims at liberating the inner self, not into some mystical state of isolation, but into oneness with others.

Yoga works to open people up mentally as well as physically. While they expand the chest and free the diaphragm to improve breathing, they also open the mind and free the personality from its self-imposed barriers. Yoga is not competitive and that alone removes impediments to communication. Yoga encourages people to become genuinely interested in others without suspecting their motives. It nurtures a sense of unity and encourages relating and sharing.

Teachers emphasize compassion, but not the superficial impulse that prompts people to feel sorry for anyone who seems less fortunate than themselves. This is not really sympathy – it is often accompanied by a smug feeling of superiority, a glimmer of satisfaction that misfortune has struck someone else. It is harmful to the sympathizer and to the object of the sympathy. Lack of compassion is also behind the tendency some people have to overcommunicate. Gushing words and inappropriate hugging and kissing can be seen as attempts to communicate by people who do not really empathize with other people and so do not know how to get through to them.

True compassion is the ability to communicate effectively and on an equal basis, and to share whatever is needed. Someone who suffers from blindness or who is confined to a wheelchair does not want sympathy but rather intuitive communication and sharing. Showing compassion involves accepting other people, whether

Yoga helps adults to regain the physical spontaneity that is natural to children.

they are of a different color or religion, whether they use sign language, or simply look sort of weird.

The greatest problem in many people's lives is a feeling of isolation. This is not necessarily loneliness, more a recurring feeling of separation from society. Children, teenagers, and old people often feel it acutely. People who feel isolated often respond by withdrawing into a shell, or developing a hard exterior, and taking up yoga is often a cry for help. Their defenses produce a chronic tension, and in the initial stages, they find yoga simply makes them feel better, because it alleviates this tension. Gradually, as the body becomes more supple, the mind becomes more receptive to the sense of unity that yoga tries to engender, and they find they no longer need to maintain their defenses.

Many of the yoga asanas incorporate gestures of openness and acceptance. These are a way of changing one's own feeling of depression or inner fear through body language. In time, these gestures become part of the natural body language from the inner self to other people. Students who have been practicing yoga for some time usually find they have loosened up in every way. Their more natural body language reflects their progressive openness, and they become more tolerant. They develop more spontaneous ways of communicating, and they feel more tactile. These changes make a difference to the way people respond to them because they are visibly at peace with themselves.

BREAKING DOWN BARRIERS

Yoga is about breaking down physical and mental barriers and passing through them. Anyone who perseveres with yoga will develop a greater closeness to other people, simply because they learn how to live without barriers, and how to perceive and dismantle the barriers created by others.

NONCOMMUNICATION

- Some people put up barriers in the form of gestures and body language as an unconscious self-protection when approached.

- Sitting with the arms folded says "You can't get at my heart."

- Noncommunicators avoid all contact with strangers.

- Competition closes people up. "Me vs. you."

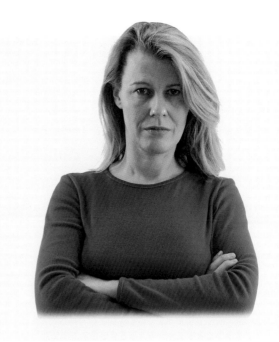

COMMUNICATION

- Yoga develops a sensitivity to other people's feelings and a genuine interest in them.

- Body language becomes naturally open, and tactile at appropriate moments.

- Yoga encourages people to have confidence in their inner selves. The result is greater openness.

- Yoga encourages a noncompetitive spirit. People are genuinely encouraging.

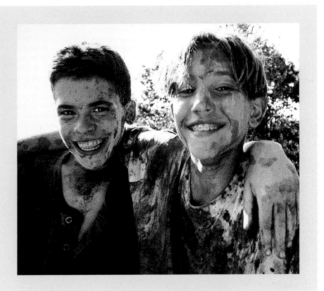

OVERCOMMUNICATION

- Gushers try too hard to communicate. They are insensitive to the reactions of other people and pretend a closeness that does not exist.

- Kissing and hugging people who are not really close devalues the meaning of close body contact.

- Forcing your attention on people reveals a lack of awareness of how they feel.

- Overcommunication can be a form of competition. Many people "collect" friends to show others how popular or well-connected they are.

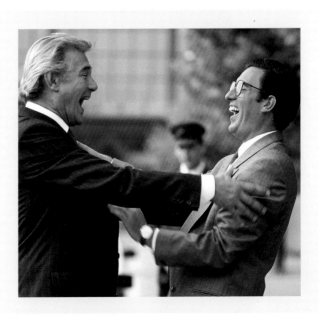

151

You Are What You Eat

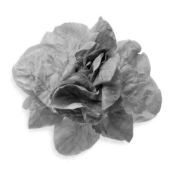

Yoga perceives eating and drinking as two ways in which prana, the Life Force, enters the human body from outside. Food and drink are therefore directly related to energy levels and spiritual awareness. Health, vitality, and mental alertness are influenced by the nature and quality of the food we eat. However, the yoga sages emphasized the middle path in food and drink as in other aspects of living, counseling against eating (and drinking) too little or too much.

Many interpretations have been made of the guidelines on diet in the ancient yoga texts. Some are very pedantic, giving precise rules for the number of times each mouthful of food must be chewed before swallowing. In essence, however, what the major yoga texts recommend is maintaining a balance in eating. "Eat sensibly" is their advice, and they impose few rules.

Yoga has always been closely associated with vegetarianism, perhaps because of India's ancient Hindu beliefs, for climatic reasons, or because of an attitude of nonviolence toward animals. Yoga considers vegetarian food wholesome, but it does not rule out eating fish or meat. Humans have flourished because they are omnivorous; the body is designed to survive on an astonishingly wide diet. Vegetarianism is, in fact, a side issue in yoga and not something that points along the path to samadhi.

Some people come to regard food as a panacea for all their ills, from mood swings to weight imbalances and symptoms of illness. If changing their diet does not work, they may take up yoga to try to deal with what they see as their problems. Yoga is not a therapy, however, and its response is to ignore the specific complaints of such students and encourage them to work holistically on strengthening the control of the senses (see pages 148–49). Students who respond find this approach very beneficial.

Through mind control yoga does gradually influence the impulse to eat. As students gain control over their senses and begin to feel more peaceful, they may gradually become more discriminating about their food. They may begin to eat more regularly, drink less alcohol, or feel more inclined toward eating healthier food, such as vegetables and fruit, rather than processed foods or precooked meals. At this point they may begin to read about diet. Those who feel they are too fat find that learning to control the mind makes it easier to follow a diet.

After overindulging in some annual festival, such as Christmas, to spend 24 hours without eating, just drinking fruit juice every two hours, allows the digestive system to recover its equilibrium. But longer-term fasting has no value in yoga. The heightened consciousness that fasting is said to produce is due to no more than pathological changes in the electrochemical balance, and is of no benefit. Moderation in everything is the way of yoga.

It is best not to eat just before yoga practice, but a glass of fruit juice up to half an hour beforehand will do no harm.

MEALTIMES AND YOGA PRACTICE

It is unwise to eat shortly before practicing yoga because the process of digestion diverts blood and energy from the rest of the body. The table below gives guidelines on how long to leave between eating or drinking and yoga practice. Note that the stomach should be empty before practicing the uddiyana bandha (see pages 106–7) because it puts great pressure on the abdomen.

TYPE OF MEAL	TIME TO LEAVE BEFORE PRACTICE	TYPE OF PRACTICE
all	4 hours	abdominal stretches and massage
heavy	2 hours	all stretches and asanas
light	1 hour	asanas
snack	1 hour	all stretches and asanas
nonalcoholic drink	½ hour	all stretches and asanas

WHAT THE SAGES RECOMMEND

Sattvic foods are described in the Bhavagad Gita as those that promote life, vitality, strength, health, joy, and cheerfulness. They are what we think of as "healthy eating" – most important are the "good grains": rice, barley, and wheat; dairy foods; honey, ginger, cucumber, and leafy vegetables, and clean water. Consuming neither too little nor too much, and eating a widely varied diet may still be the best rules to follow, however.

Vegetarian diets need pulses and grains to provide first-class protein.

Rajasic foods are said to be bitter, sour, salty, very hot, pungent, and harsh, and they produce grief, pain, and disease. Translated into modern terms, they are foods that have lost their nutrient value: they have dried out, or have been reheated and have become contaminated. Too many condiments, such as salt, relishes, and mustards, are thought to reduce the nutrient value of many foods.

Beware the hidden dangers in tempting nibbles like chips and chocolate, too much spice and endless cups of coffee.

Tamasic foods are spoilt, tasteless, putrid, stale, and unclean. They have been adulterated with preservatives and artificial color and flavor, precooked and prepacked, poor imitations of the real foods the body needs. The healthiest food is uncontaminated with chemical pesticides and additives, so eating organically grown cereal grains, fresh vegetables, fruit, and dairy foods is sensible.

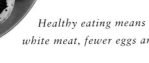

Healthy eating means more fish and fresh white meat, fewer eggs and less preserved meat.

You Are What You Think

In recent years it has become a generally accepted fact that the interaction between our thoughts and our physical body affects our energy and our health. Yet this idea is far from new. It was first expressed some 2,500 years ago, when the Buddha declared, "You are what you think."

The basis of human life is self-awareness. Between rising in the morning and falling asleep, people constantly relate themselves to what is going on around them. Through the senses, this awareness penetrates the body and is carried as nerve impulses from eyes, ears, and skin sensors to the brain, and from the brain to other parts of the body. This is what stimulates the impulse to sleep in the dark and the impetus to awaken in daylight. Thus, nerve impulses connect every cell in the body to the brain and, through the nervous system, to the immune system.

All the body's functions, from brainwaves to heart beat, from breathing to energy flow, have a rhythm, and all the body's rhythms interrelate. As thoughts are released from the brain they may harmonize with this interplay of rhythms, or they may disturb the pattern. An anxiety may send a discordant note through the body, and if that continues, a counterflow develops against the body's natural, calm rhythm. That is the point at which people begin to wonder why they feel tired, why this pain has started.

Every thought is related directly to the immune system, and while one stray thought will not produce illness, recurrent negative images that develop into a habit of thought may become the precursor to disease. Yoga tries to free the body rhythms from jarring counterflows so that nothing interferes with their natural harmony. It works to calm the mind, so the body functions better. It is important, however, not to become fixated on the asanas and neglect the spirit. Some people learn to execute a whole program of asanas, yet still lack inner stillness.

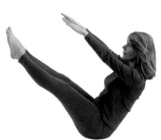

It is essential to maintain a balance in yoga and not to become too absorbed in perfecting the asanas.

Anyone who practices yoga needs to learn from the beginning how to develop a sense of stillness. It involves setting aside just five minutes at the end of each practice to rest, develop a steady breathing rhythm, and quieten the mind. At first it may seem a chore, but it is vital to persist. It soon becomes a pleasing interval to look forward to instead. Gradually, it develops into a heartfelt need and once that point is reached, harmony and healing can begin.

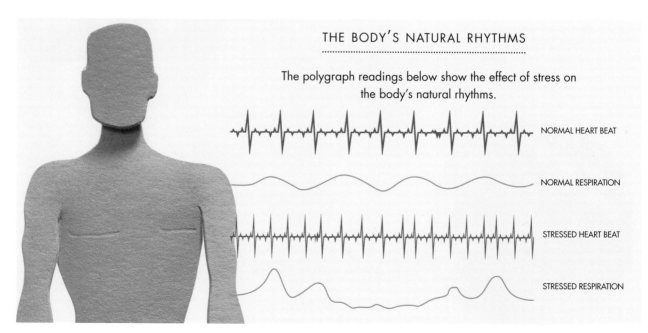

THE BODY'S NATURAL RHYTHMS

The polygraph readings below show the effect of stress on the body's natural rhythms.

NORMAL HEART BEAT

NORMAL RESPIRATION

STRESSED HEART BEAT

STRESSED RESPIRATION

CREATING HARMONY

The body can adjust to temporary strains, but a state of permanent tension causes damage and illness. Tension is not always easy to detect, but breathing is an excellent indication of how relaxed the body is. Work on creating inner calm by dedicating yourself to daily breathing practice. At other times, try to remember to stop now and again and try to relieve your body tension. Be calm and peaceful as often as you can, and use meditation to bring about true internal stillness and harmony.

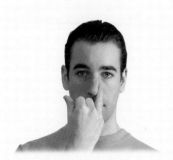

Breathing

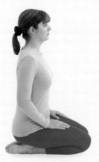

Meditation

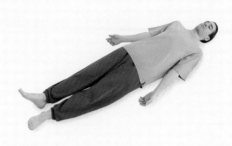

Relaxation

RELEASING SUPPRESSED ANGER

Yoga explores the link between mind and body to deal with negative thinking, depression, and momentary irritation or frustration. The mind can be tricked into a happier state simply by smiling, making the whole body feel better.

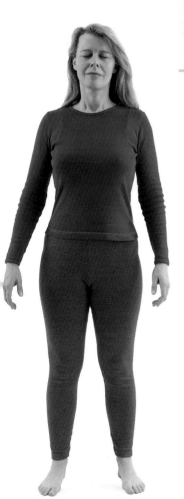

1 *The moment you become conscious that your feelings are low, sit or stand erect, balance your head, look straight ahead, place your hands on your thighs or at your sides, and breathe rhythmically for a few seconds. The sense of depression or annoyance will soon begin to fade.*

2 *On an in-breath, raise your hands and arms sideways into the air until they form an upward arc. By making this gesture of exultation, you force your negative feelings to assume their correct perspective. Repeat the movement several times, until you feel like smiling, and do it whenever such feelings threaten to return.*

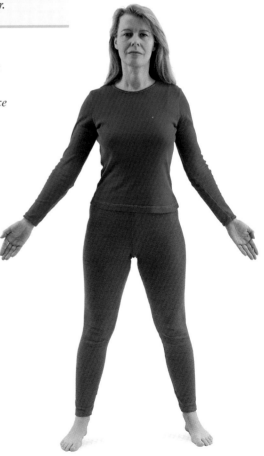

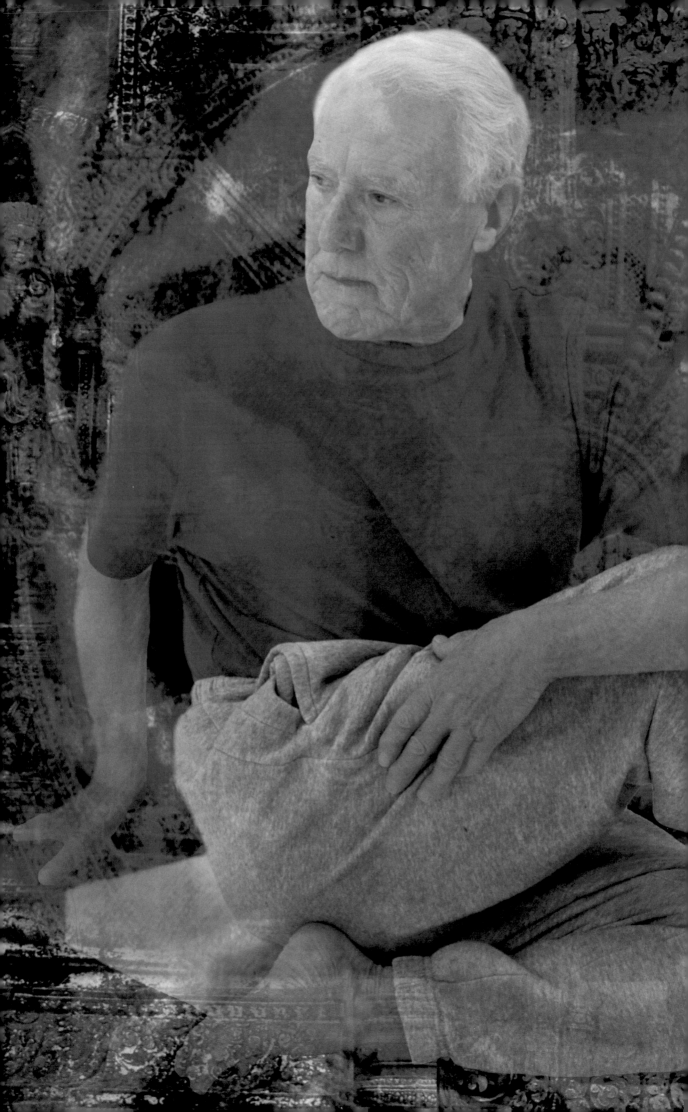

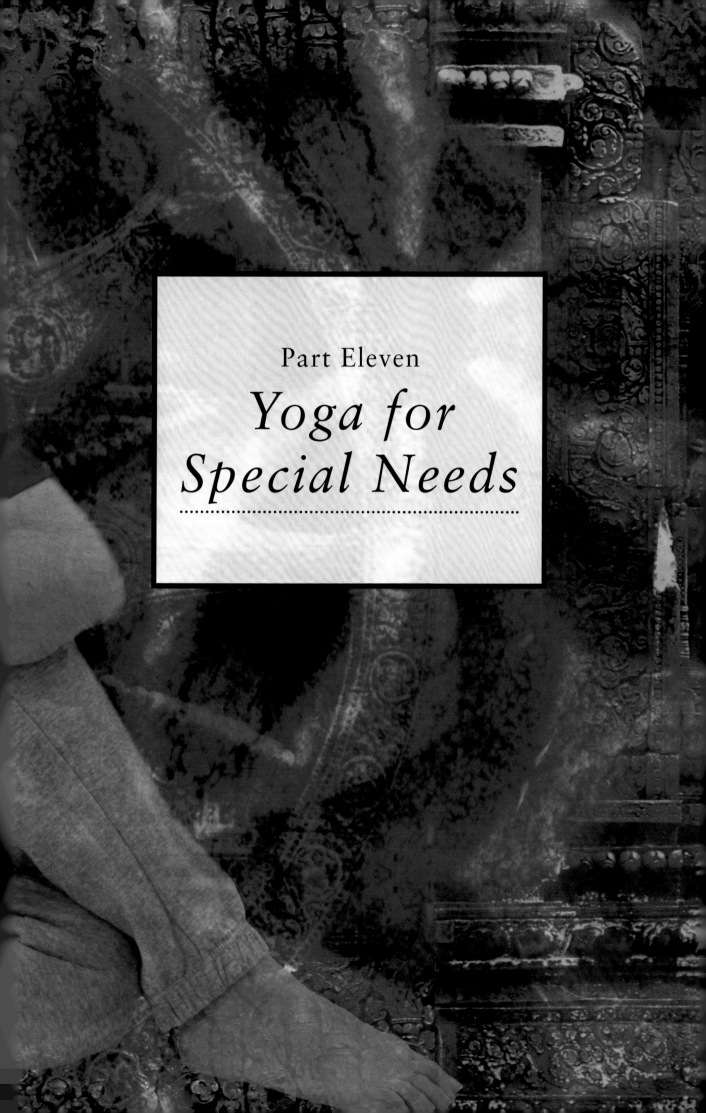

Part Eleven

*Yoga for
Special Needs*

Special Needs

....

Yoga is of benefit to everyone throughout their life, but in its long history there have been many yoga teachers who, seeing the help that yoga could give to particular groups, dedicated themselves to exploring ways in which it could answer their special needs.

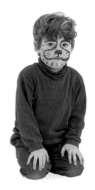

Young children can benefit from yoga.

For more than 20 years teachers at the Yoga for Health Foundation have investigated the role of yoga in helping people with special needs. They have explored ways of teaching yoga to children from the age of five to the teenage years, to old people, and to women during pregnancy. They have gained worldwide recognition for their work on the role of yoga in relieving and combating illness (see pages 170–71), and they have pioneered ways of teaching yoga to people with disabilities.

One of the aims of yoga is helping people to realize the full potential of their mind and body. This aim applies to people with limbs that cannot function properly or with uncoordinated movements. In many cases yoga cannot restore function to the affected area of the body, but through stretching, breathing, and specially adapted asanas, it can overcome some of the problems disablement causes by restoring full function to the rest of the body. It can teach a body tensed with frustration to relax, and by retraining the lungs to breathe normally, it can reach parts of the mind and body that may have been neglected for years.

No one is too young or too old to start yoga. Mothers can take their babies to postnatal yoga classes, and teach their children simple animal poses to maintain their natural suppleness. If the body is gently stretched and exercised during pregnancy it will recover its former shape and elasticity more quickly. Yoga prepares it for labor, and is an ideal postnatal exercise. Mothers who continue yoga after pregnancy may find that prolapse, incontinence, osteoporosis and other problems of later life do not occur.

The following pages give guidelines for disabled people, children, pregnant women, and older people, all of whom have special needs. For more specialist information and advice, refer to the booklist on pages 184–85, or contact the Yoga for Health Foundation, whose address is given on page 182.

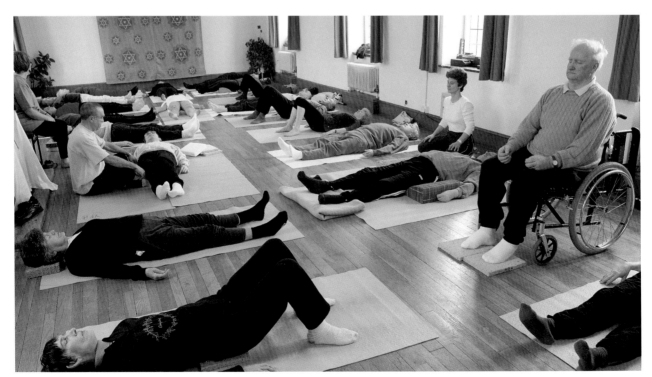

The Yoga for Health Foundation runs special needs classes for people with many different disabilities.

YOGA FOR ALL

Many older people find yoga helps them maintain mobility into old age, while others find that progressive yoga exercises help them restore mobility to parts of the body that have stiffened through neglect. Regular yoga practice prevents many illnesses of later life.

People with disabilities are not ill and benefit from hatha yoga in the same way as people with the ability to walk and run. Yoga is an excellent way to exercise for anyone who spends much of their time in a wheelchair.

Pregnant women find gentle stretching and breathing prepares their bodies for labor and helps them keep in shape so they recover quickly from late pregnancy and delivery. These days, many mothers take their infants to postnatal mother-and-baby classes.

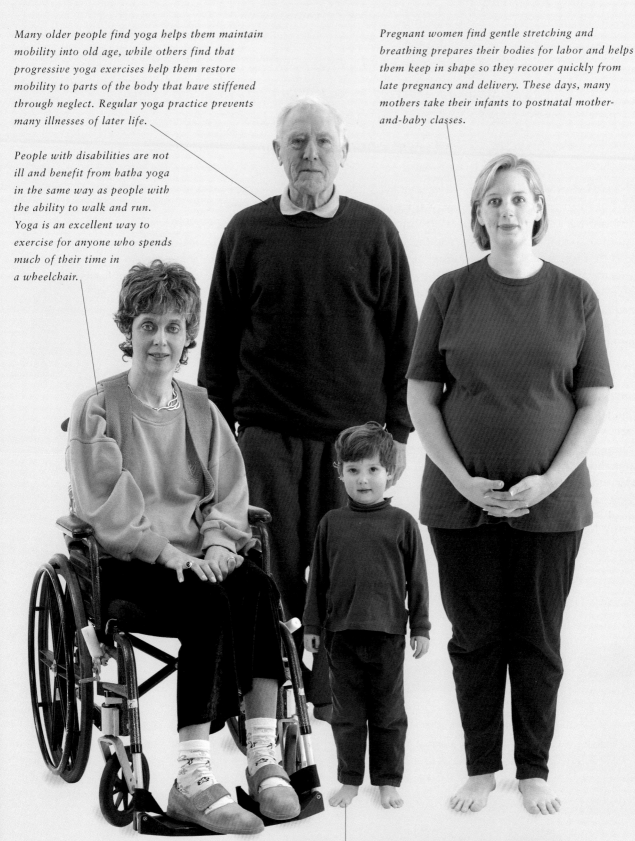

Children aged from 4–5 can attend yoga classes. Stretching and exercise helps them maintain their natural suppleness. Learning the value of effective breathing and relaxation can help them during their teenage years and into adulthood.

Working with Disabilities and Injuries

There is no special yoga for people with disabilities. The range of asanas is so wide that every disabled person will be able to put together an integrated program of those that seem adaptable to their circumstances.

Every person with a disability has special needs, and to benefit to the full from yoga will require some specialist advice. There are many different disabilities and their special treatment is beyond the scope of this book. But it is also true that everyone can benefit from regularly practicing the simple stretches illustrated on this page, and from the breathing, visualization, and meditation techniques illustrated elsewhere.

Yoga is not a substitute for physiotherapy, so if in doubt about whether to try out an asana, it is a good idea to ask a trusted physician, nurse or physiotherapist for advice. It is sensible to begin with the simplest movements. These are not only practical and adaptable for disabled people, they also produce surprising improvements. Prolonged sitting in a wheelchair or walking with a stick can make sitting upright difficult, so practice sitting or standing erect in front of a mirror, and work on developing a rhythmic breathing pattern. The feeling of mental wellbeing improved posture brings is a welcome bonus.

PRACTICING GOOD POSTURE

If you have a disability or perhaps a temporary injury that has affected one side, standing upright can be a difficult feat, so practice standing and taking steps while keeping your body as erect as you can. Check whether you are standing upright by doing the wall test (see page 63). Ask other people whether you are sitting upright. If possible, practice the asanas in front of a mirror to make sure you are not doing them in a lopsided way.

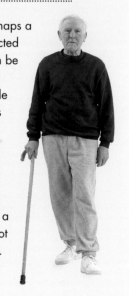

STRETCHING WHILE LYING DOWN

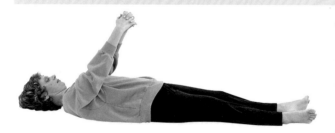

Finding solutions to problems is part of being human. If you are not able to stand to stretch, you can get around this by stretching while lying on the floor. You can exercise the feet, legs, arms, free the head and neck, and stretch the whole body while lying on your back.

1 *Lie on your back with your feet together and your arms by your side, palms down. Breathe out and as you breathe in, slowly lift your arms, stretching them, until the back of your hands touch the floor behind your head.*

2 *Extend your whole body, pulling your toes downward and your fingers upward. Breathe out slowly, then gradually stretch your arms back to your sides. Relax and repeat several times. Stretching like this every day will aid your posture as well as giving you a sense of well-being.*

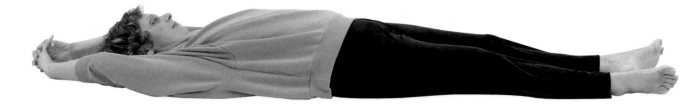

EXERCISING ON WHEELS

*Wheelchair users need to work out ways of adapting the
asanas to fit their special circumstances. Here is one
solution to performing a forward bend in a chair instead
of sitting on the floor. You will immediately feel the
benefit of stretching the whole of your spine from your
lower back to your neck.*

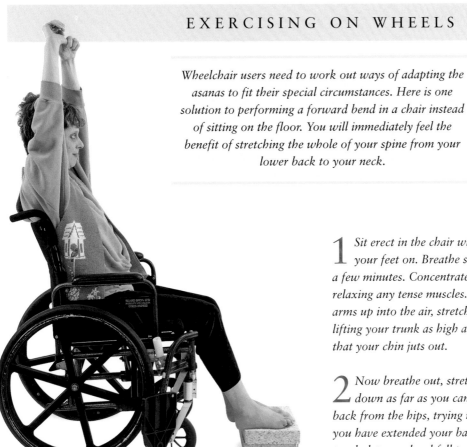

1 Sit erect in the chair with some foam blocks to rest
your feet on. Breathe slowly and deeply in and out for
a few minutes. Concentrate on your body, contracting and
relaxing any tense muscles. On an in-breath, swing your
arms up into the air, stretching them over your head and
lifting your trunk as high as you can. Raise your head so
that your chin juts out.

2 Now breathe out, stretching your arms forward and
down as far as you can. As you do so, stretch your
back from the hips, trying not to bend your trunk. When
you have extended your back as far as you can, bend your
trunk, let your head fall toward your thighs, and hold the
furthest comfortable part of your legs – your shins, ankles,
or feet. Hold the stretch for up to half a minute, breathing
in and out.

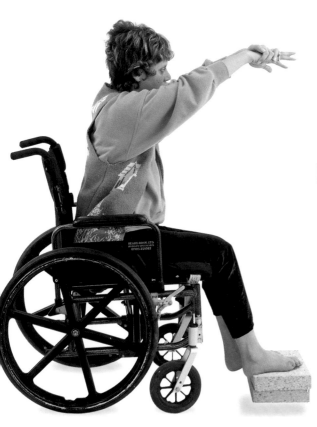

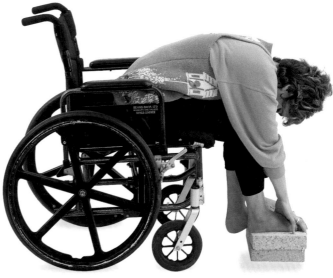

3 On an in-breath, slowly sit up, swinging your arms into
the air, then lowering them to your sides. Relax and
breathe normally for a few minutes, then repeat steps 1 and
2, trying to hold the stretch for up to two minutes.

Yoga for Pregnancy

·······································

As long as you choose the right exercises, yoga makes an excellent preparation for childbirth. Stretches and asanas keep the body supple and strong and the spine erect. Relaxation and meditation alleviate many of the common disorders of pregnancy, from back pain to high blood pressure, and breathing is an invaluable preparation for labor.

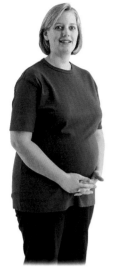

Many yoga asanas prepare the body for labor.

During the first three months of pregnancy there is always a danger of miscarriage. This is not a good time for anyone who has never done yoga to begin practicing asanas, although gentle stretching is not harmful, and breathing and relaxation can only do good. By the beginning of the fourth month, however, it is safe to begin practicing yoga.

It is important to listen to the body and to stop if there seems any risk of overstretching the abdomen. As pregnancy advances the abdominal muscles are greatly extended and should not be stretched further, so after the third month, asanas such as the cobra should not be attempted. A gentle backward stretch is possible, however, if the back is bent over a stable support made of pillows. Exercises to increase spinal mobility are especially beneficial, since back pain is common during late pregnancy. The cat (see page 86), which exercises the spine but puts no pressure on the abdomen, is ideal, even during the later months.

Breathing and relaxation are particularly important because they can be used to reduce discomfort during labor. Women who have a long-established habit of effective breathing through yoga are better able to make use of it in labor than those who first practice breathing in prenatal classes. Breath retention exercises (see pages 118–19) can harm the fetus and should never be attempted during pregnancy.

GENTLE TWIST

The spine is forced out of alignment during pregnancy and needs to be exercised to keep it mobile and strong. It is unwise to try to perform a full twist, but this gentle twist is ideal for maintaining good posture and spinal flexibility, and it will alleviate back pain. You can adapt this exercise to suit your condition as your pregnancy advances.

3 *Hold the outside of your left knee with your right hand. Turn to the left, toward the bent knee.*

4 *Breathing normally, hold the position for up to two minutes, then relax.*

5 *Repeat steps 2 and 3, bending the right leg and holding your right knee with your left hand.*

1 *Sit comfortably erect with your legs together and extended in front of you.*

2 *Bend the left knee, so that your foot is flat on the floor, then gently move your heel back toward your thigh as far as you can.*

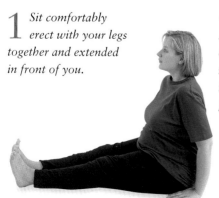

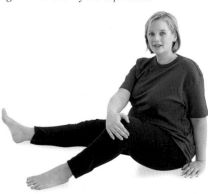

PELVIC FLOOR EXERCISES

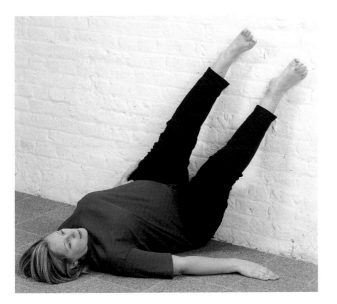

The pelvic floor muscles, which form a figure 8 around the anus and the vagina, take a lot of strain during pregnancy and labor, so exercises to stretch and strengthen them need to be carried out once a day at least. The benefits are lifelong. If these muscles are damaged and weakened during pregnancy, a weak bladder and rectum result, which can cause incontinence and even prolapse (the sagging of the womb or rectum) in later life.

1 Lie on your back with your legs straight and your heels touching a wall. Your arms should be spread out at your sides. Moving from the hips, slide your legs gently from side to side.

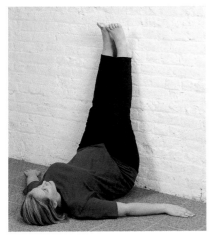

2 Return your legs to the upright position again, with your feet together and your heels resting against the wall.

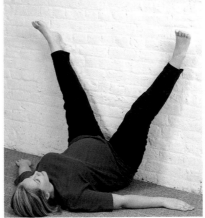

3 Keeping your heels in contact with the wall, slide your feet slowly sideways until your legs are wide apart. Hold this position, breathing normally, for up to five minutes, then slide your legs together again.

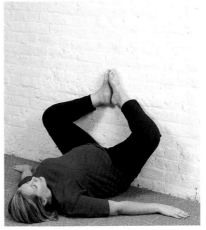

4 Bend your knees outward until you can press the soles of your feet together. Hold this position for a moment and then place the soles of your feet against the wall and relax before rising.

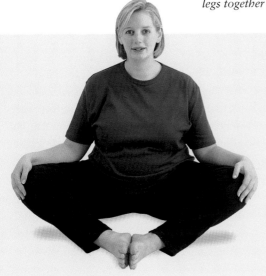

THIG MUSCLE STRETCH

1 Sit comfortably erect with your legs together and your knees bent.

2 Push your knees outward as far as you can while pressing the soles of your feet together.

3 Breathing normally, hold the position for up to five minutes, then raise your knees and place the soles of your feet on the floor.

Yoga for Children

Children find yoga fun. They have great powers of visualization, so they enter into the spirit of being a cobra or a cat, hissing and wriggling as they raise their heads, purring with contentment as they arch their backs. Ask them to imitate a tree and they will stand for minutes, stretching up, surprisingly silent and able to be still.

Yoga can be good for children aged from 4 or 5 years onward, although it not advisable to begin before that age because up to then the bones are still very soft and could be damaged. The bones continue to grow into the late teens, so children should not be pushed into complex asanas and spinal twists, but rather encouraged to explore their bodies' natural flexibility. Simple exercises will do children no harm and early training in good posture and effective breathing, with movements that gently stretch and exercise the muscles, can prevent damage and immobility in later life.

By stimulating their imaginative powers during exercise, yoga encourages natural relationships between body and mind that can be more difficult to nurture later in life. Being able to relax effectively at will is as important for children, to help them deal with the stresses of daily life, as it is for adults. It is an invaluable skill that, once it becomes a habit, will be with them all their lives.

While younger children are usually extremely flexible, finding it natural to sit in the lotus position, for instance, some teenagers seem to go through a stiff and awkward phase, characterized by bad posture and a shying away from physical exercise. The reason may be partly psychological. Not only are teenagers growing fast but they are also moving away from the comfort and simplicity of their childhood realities into a different and more complicated adult world. Acne, mood changes, and other body and mind disorders are symptoms of the resulting stress. Yoga can do a great deal to alleviate these problems by restoring flexibility and maintaining balanced movement through gentle stretching and deep relaxation. It encourages teenagers to be proud of their bodies rather than ashamed of them, and to realize exactly what they can do.

Yoga teachers continually explore new frontiers. Recently, academics in the West have been experimenting with yoga sessions that mothers and their infants can participate in together. During the 1990s Dr. Françoise Freedman, a British social anthropologist, began yoga courses for mothers and babies – some only six months old. The babies seem to benefit especially from their mothers' deep relaxation, and it may be that children pick up signals from their mothers' breathing patterns, so that when mothers become more relaxed, their children respond, becoming quieter and perhaps altering their breathing pattern.

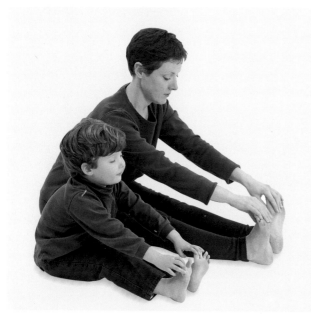

MOTHER AND CHILD YOGA

When mothers and their children practice yoga together, both benefit. In mother-and-baby yoga sessions mothers hold their infants while practicing asanas, reaching out to them during posterior stretches, for example, and leaning toward them during forward bends. The babies appear to respond to these activities and to be happier and less fractious afterward. Toddlers enjoy doing simple stretches and try to copy what their mothers do. They join in the breathing practice and seem to respond to relaxation sessions, lying quietly on the floor in the corpse pose, apparently relaxing too.

BEING A LION

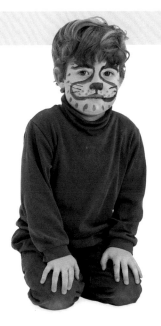

Even when they are in a dangerous situation, being threatened and having to defend their cubs, lions always take time to get their bodies in line before they attack. If their spine is not straight or their head is down, their attack will be weaker. When they are ready, they put all the force of their body and their mind into roaring and being threatening, so their frightened opponent will be scared off and run away.

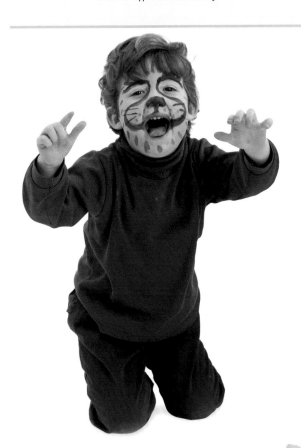

1 Kneel on the mat and sit back on your heels. Now shake your back and shoulders to remove the tension from your muscles, and sit up, trying to make your spine longer. Nod your head to check that it feels properly balanced. Rest your hands on your knees and look straight ahead.

2 Now breathe in deeply through your nose and think hard about attacking. Open your mouth as wide as you can and breathe out fast, shouting "Ha!" so the air is forced out. Stick your tongue right out and bend it right down so it touches your chin. Glare at your nosetip. Raise your hands and tighten all the muscles in your arms, hands, and fingers.

3 Let all your muscles relax slowly, and sit as you were before. Breathe normally for a few minutes, then practice being a lion again. This time, really imagine you are a lion and make yourself as ferocious as you can.

A MIND GAME

Find a tray and put it on a table, then go out of the room and ask another person to put as many small objects on the tray as will fit. You must not see what objects are collected and put on the tray. Find some paper and a pencil, and when the tray is full stand in front of it and look at all the objects on it. Try to remember as many as you can. Now sit somewhere where you cannot see the tray and write down all the objects you can remember, taking no more than five minutes. After that, go back and see how many you got right.

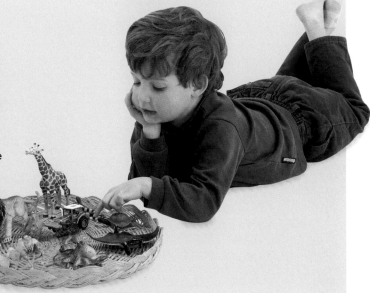

Yoga for the Elderly

People who have practiced yoga all their lives continue to do so into old age. Yoga teachers in their nineties can assume with ease postures that still elude students more than 70 years their junior. One outstanding example is Indra Devi, a Russian-born yoga teacher who celebrated her 100th birthday in 1999.

Western medicine has made little effort to investigate the physical potential of older bodies. Yoga has never been guilty of such neglect. Teachers have always encouraged older people to practice, to use stretching and relaxation to keep muscles flexible and the spine and joints mobile. Posture and breathing alone will help counteract the stiffening effects of a sedentary life. Body and mind can never be disassociated, and older people who fear their memory is failing them often find that effective breathing, practiced regularly, restores it to its former efficiency.

People who begin yoga in the last decades of their life must set themselves to achieve what they are capable of, and not aim at the impossible. For instance, at first they may need to spend days relearning simply to stand erect, or, if it seems impossible to sit on the floor, working on the spine while sitting in a chair or lying on the floor. It is important to listen to the body and heed its warnings about how far it is able to go. At the same time, it is essential not to be held back by imaginary limitations. Just because something takes time does not mean it cannot be achieved. The secret is to explore gently, but never to give up exploring.

Mind and body work together, and one thing yoga does is restore the confidence in the human body that negative Western attitudes to aging help to erode. Above all, people in their sixties and older need to be aware of the tremendous range of movement of which their bodies are capable. This student has been practicing yoga for many years and executes a perfect twist with ease.

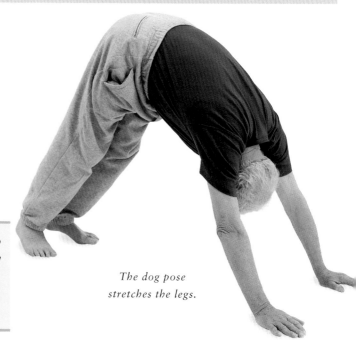

Yoga is a lifelong activity and is not restricted to the young and fit.

CAT AND DOG

The cat pose stretches the back and abdomen.

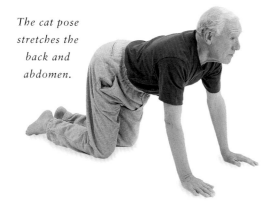

The simpler spinal exercises are intended for people who have back problems or who have not exercised for many years. If you are fairly supple, the cat and dog poses illustrated on pages 86–87 help make the muscles of the spine and trunk more mobile.

The dog pose stretches the legs.

WORKING ON THE BACK

The stiffening of the back is a common problem among older people. Begin slowly and cautiously – sudden vigorous exercise will only damage the spine. The back will respond, however, to these gentle mobility exercises if they are carried out every day. Correct breathing and deep relaxation after each practice session are as important as the exercise.

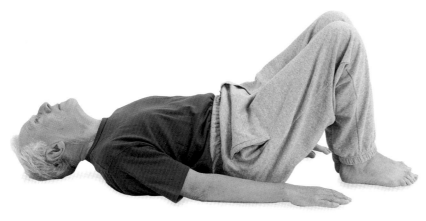

1 *Lie on the floor with your hands by your sides. Spend a few minutes breathing in and out, concentrating on relaxing any tense muscles. When you are ready, bend your knees, bringing your heels as close as you can to your hips. Your knees should be touching.*

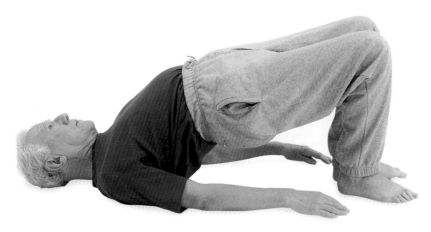

2 *Breathe out slowly while trying to lift your buttocks off the floor. Do this by tensing the muscles of your thighs and your lower abdomen, and tilting your pelvis upward. If you find it difficult, do not try to raise your back; instead, press your palms against the ground.*

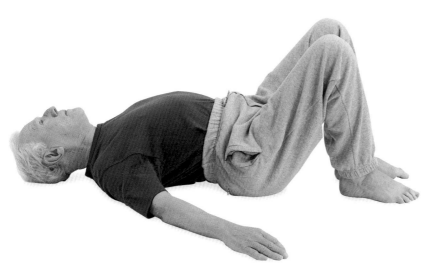

3 *Breathing in, lower your buttocks to the floor and arch your back, resting your weight on your buttocks and your shoulders. Breathe out and relax. Repeat steps 1 and 2 several times in succession, concentrating on creating a rocking movement and thinking about your breathing.*

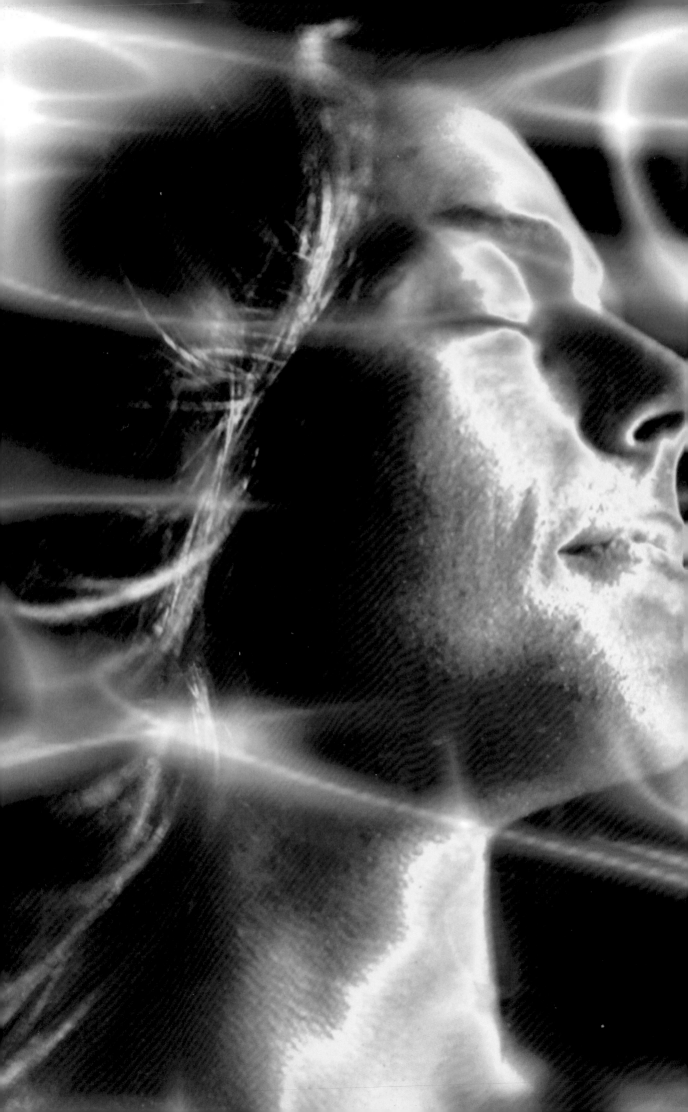

Part Twelve

Yoga and Healing

Healing

·················

Yoga is not a therapy, but it has an important therapeutic role: there can be no illness upon which it will not have a beneficial effect. It is a holistic system, so regards illnesses as symptoms of some imbalance between mind and body. Yoga is concerned with discovering how to assist the body to correct its own imbalance, and, in the process, clear up the symptoms of illness.

A letter from a Scottish physiotherapist wanting to know whether yoga could help people with multiple sclerosis was the impetus that led to the formation of the Yoga for Health Foundation during the 1970s. The therapeutic role of yoga has since been shown with courses aimed at combating multiple sclerosis and ME, arthritis, asthma, and even cancer are held at its residential center in southern England.

After an injury, deep breathing will stimulate the circulation of blood and tissue fluid. These carry blood-clotting substances, cells that fight infection, and electrically charged

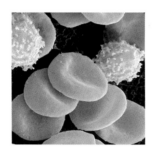

White cells circulate among the red cells in the blood, attacking invading foreign cells.

chemical particles called electrolytes, to the injury site for repair. Tensions set up in the body by the injury affect the blood flow, causing blockages in small blood vessels. Deep relaxation extends right down to these tiny capillaries, easing them so blood can circulate through them.

Through its unique relationship with the consciousness, yoga also stimulates the body's immune system, strengthening its power to prevent illness as well as its ability to repair injury and combat disease. The following pages explore some of the many ways in which yoga can help fight illness and maintain health.

BANISHING THE BLUES

The link between mind and body is clearly shown in the aftermath of illness. Pain, loss of mobility, or simply the sense that you are out of the swim of things can lead to a sense of despondency, which makes recovery more difficult.

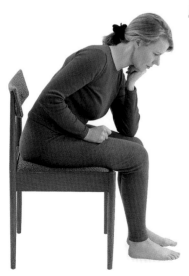

1 *Conscious action can help to overcome an attack of the blues, whether associated with illness or not. Slumping miserably prevents you from breathing deeply, and can lead to hyperventilation as your body attempts to increase the supply of oxygen.*

2 *Make a conscious effort to sit correctly with your spine erect and your hands resting on your thighs. This will allow deeper and more controlled breathing. It is also difficult to maintain your miserable outloook in this position.*

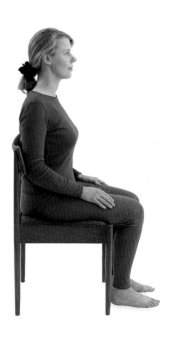

THE ELECTROMAGNETIC SYSTEM

Yoga always held that breathing helps maintain health by stimulating the body's electrical systems, but not until scientists investigated electricity did physiologists understand its role in the body. They found that tiny electrical impulses are generated by neurons or nerve cells and carried along their extensions – the axons or nerves – to junctions called synapses. Here, neurotransmitter chemicals transmit them to nearby neurons. The cell body is surrounded by branchlike dendrites that also transmit neurotransmitter chemicals. The dendrites pick up impulses from neighboring neurons and carry them toward the cell body. In this way impulses are sent to and from the brain. Electrical impulses govern the heart beat and have an important role in repairing bone injuries.

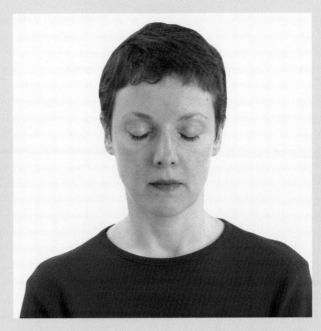

Relaxation and concentrating on your breathing will help speed the healing process.

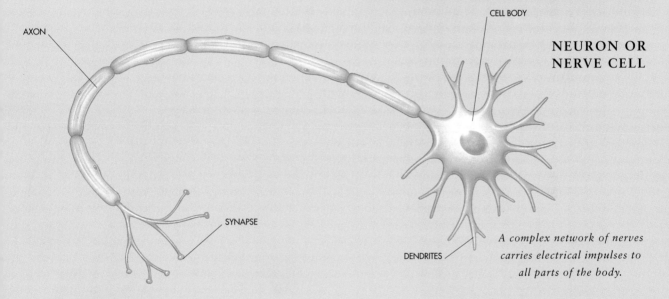

AXON

CELL BODY

NEURON OR NERVE CELL

SYNAPSE

DENDRITES

A complex network of nerves carries electrical impulses to all parts of the body.

Every cell in the body is bathed in tissue fluid. It consists mainly of water and dissolved oxygen, carbon dioxide, and other nutrients, and circulates in the blood and lymph. When a cell requires nutrients, its surrounding membrane allows selected molecules to pass through. Circulating in the tissue fluid are electrolytes. These are chemicals such as sodium, potassium, magnesium, and calcium that can split into positive and negative ions (electrically charged particles) when dissolved in fluid, and one of their essential roles in the body is to effect the transmission of electrical impulses along nerves. The body carefully controls its levels of electrolytes, and low concentrations indicate disease.

Right: *In a two-way exchange, water molecules, electrolytes, and nutrients, such as oxygen carried by red blood cells, pass through the walls of blood capillaries and tissue cells, and chemicals from tissue cells pass back into the blood.*

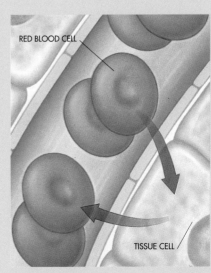

RED BLOOD CELL

TISSUE CELL

Managing Illness

Teachers who work with people experiencing illness begin by teaching yoga, just as it is set out in this book. Meanwhile, they observe, question, and listen, trying to relate the complaint to each individual. Their immediate aim is to encourage everyone to take control of their own illness, find their own ways of coping with it, and stimulate their own healing abilities.

This approach is applied to all illnesses, from a tension headache to arthritis to cancer. The way to combat colds and migraines, insomnia, and allergies is to find a way of allowing the mind to manage the illness instead of letting the illness dominate. Yoga harnesses the forces of mind and body to restore balance and reduce tension, giving the body a chance to fight back. Persistence leads to gradual progress, and in time, it is hoped, minor disorders recur less frequently and eventually fade out.

Poor posture and a sedentary life are the causes of many chronic illnesses. The abdominal organs can almost seize up as a result of unrelieved muscular tension. This can be caused by something as correctable as permanent stooping or lack of exercise; and it can be the cause of irritable bowel syndrome, colitis, and chronic constipation. Just learning to stand erect and work the diaphragm brings relief. It restores the rhythmic pressure that effective breathing exerts on the organs of the diaphragm, and gradually stimulates

their normal functioning. Symptoms such as headaches, stomach pains, and skin disorders may lessen or disappear as a result of regularly practicing some of the exercises contained in this book.

No one yet understands the causes of ME, Parkinson's disease, and multiple sclerosis, but a nervous element is a feature of all. Yoga encourages self-help, raises energy and stamina, and finds ways of reducing symptoms. People with breathing difficulties are encouraged to attempt asanas that open the chest and combat the fear of breathing. Sufferers from arthritis are encouraged to keep their limbs moving, to relax, and to use mind control to deal with pain.

Although the therapeutic use of yoga for patients with cancer is still controversial, its successful use by eminent physicians to relieve symptoms and help people strengthen their innate ability to fight illness has won wide recognition. Breathing with visualization, relaxation, and meditation techniques can help reduce pain and restore flexibility.

RELAXING INTO SLEEP

Make time to unwind before bedtime. If you eat late, drink alcohol, and rush home late you are unlikely to fall asleep quickly. Eat early and lightly, and drink little. Prepare for the next morning in a relaxed way. Some slow, gentle stretches will relieve any tension in your muscles. If you are relaxed you will sleep more deeply.

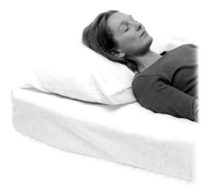

1 *Lie on your back at first. Let your breathing slow to a gentle rhythm centered in the upper part of the lungs. Continue to breathe lightly and let your mind rest on the regular rise and fall of of your breathing.*

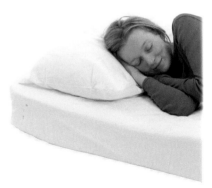

2 *Let your body find its sleeping position. Visualize an image of harmony, such as a blue sky, and concentrate on its tranquility. If you wake early, just breathe slowly and recall your images.*

MANAGING HEADACHES AND MIGRAINES

A pain in the head causes the body to tense up, and this constricts the breathing. It is thought that some migraines may stem from hyperventilation – shallow breathing – since this constricts the blood vessels to the brain. In the short term, try these measures to relieve the tension:

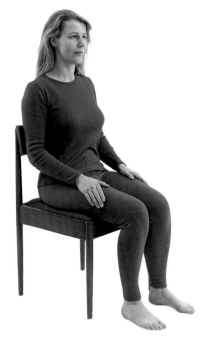

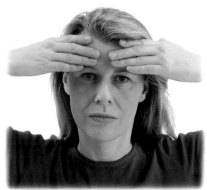

1 As you feel the headache coming on, try to find a quiet place where you can sit erect and breathe for a few minutes, establishing a gentle rhythm and concentrating on the out-breath. Think about the tension in your body and try to release it.

2 For a headache at the front of your head, rest your fingers on your forehead so the left-hand and right-hand fingertips are touching. On an in-breath, move them out to the sides, and on the out-breath, move them back together. Repeat this step several times, concentrating on the pleasant massage.

INSTANT COLD CURE

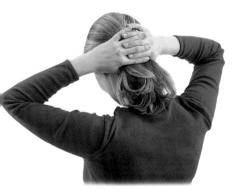

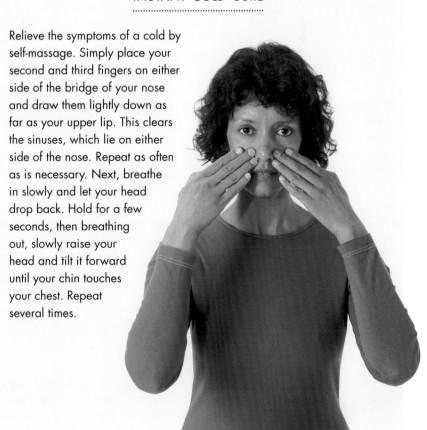

3 For a pain at the back of your head, link your fingers behind your head at the level of your ears. Breathe in, then breathe out strongly, and slowly lower your head until your chin almost touches your chest. Hold the position for a few seconds, then gradually raise your head, breathing in. Repeat several times.

Relieve the symptoms of a cold by self-massage. Simply place your second and third fingers on either side of the bridge of your nose and draw them lightly down as far as your upper lip. This clears the sinuses, which lie on either side of the nose. Repeat as often as is necessary. Next, breathe in slowly and let your head drop back. Hold for a few seconds, then breathing out, slowly raise your head and tilt it forward until your chin touches your chest. Repeat several times.

Yoga as Preventive Medicine

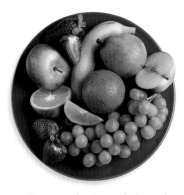

Yoga emphasizes a balanced diet to maintain health.

Practicing yoga seriously may mean making fundamental changes to one's lifestyle. It might involve reorganizing everyday life to make time for practice and meditation, eating different types of food, exploring new ways of relating to and dealing with other people, even finding a different, less stressful, type of work. The resulting new lifestyle will be a healthier one, because preventing illness is much more than taking up exercise and practicing breathing: it is a way of life.

Genetics and poor nutrition, pollution and unhygienic living conditions all cause ill health, but equal contributions are made by uncontrolled drinking, smoking, and eating, and overdependence on tranquilizers and antidepressants. Unceasing hurry causes illness and accidents, as does relentless pressure at work or in the home. Cities and rural areas, and the highways that run through them, are full of people at different stages of irritation, annoyance, and rage. In the end, the effect of all these factors on the mind and body is illness.

The body's ability to cure itself of injury and disease is easy to see, but its miraculous powers to prevent itself from becoming ill are less visible. The immune system is one known example, and medical science is rapidly discovering more. Yoga teaches that the body's self-healing systems do not work in isolation but together, and all involve the mind. The yogic approach to preventing illness is to explore ways of encouraging body and mind to work in symbiosis to remain well, resting on the firm belief that prevention is far better than cure. One important technique used is the stimulation of the electromagnetic system through breathing in order to support and strengthen the body's natural immune system.

Every body has its own strengths and weaknesses, and every body's owner is its most effective healer. The way to prevent illness is to find out what the body's needs are and how to supply them by experimenting with its response to different yoga techniques. Try to recognize personal problem areas and concentrate on tailoring a yogic regime to best suited to your needs. People prone to overindulgence in food or drugs might find that meditation gradually relieves their craving. Those who know they are susceptible to heart disease might concentrate on relaxation and breathing, and those likely to develop osteoporosis (bone loss) need lots of gentle stretching and deep-breathing practice.

It is important to practice mind contol and learn how to remain dispassionate about the prospect of disease, aging, and even death. Although it is only natural to think about such things from time to time, becoming obsessive about preventing illness is to invite tension, and that is the best way of becoming ill.

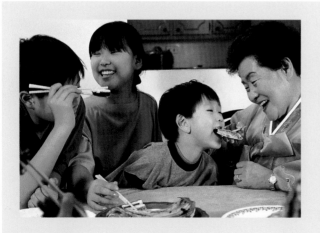

SHARING

The immune system is affected by negative emotions such as depression, grief, and isolation. Sharing is the most effective antidote to feeling low, and it is now generally accepted that it plays an important role in preventing the immune system from becoming ineffective and allowing the body to succumb to disease. Psychiatrists, physicians, and yoga teachers all know that feelings of grief, loneliness, and failure are lessened by sharing them with family and friends; and that illness is less likely among people who spend time sharing love and laughter.

VISUALIZATION

This technique creates a strong sense of harmony between mind and body. It takes practice to achieve full concentration, but it can help to visualize a still object that suggests harmony, such as a rose, or a cloud in a blue sky. Visualization is successful when it creates a feeling of stillness, so that the breathing slows and becomes regular and rhythmic. Regular visualization sessions stimulate the immune system.

MEDITATION

Among many changes that take place in the body during meditation, the breathing slows from some 15–17 breaths a minute to perhaps 6, and the amount of oxygen used declines by about 10 percent. In recent years skeptical Western physicians and surgeons have come to accept the healing effects of meditation. Yoga teaches that by relaxing into a state of total physical and mental peace, energy is conserved and allowed to flow freely, stimulating the body systems, such as blood flow. The circulation of blood in the muscles increases by up to 300 percent during meditation. Like sleep, meditation allows the body's healing systems to operate.

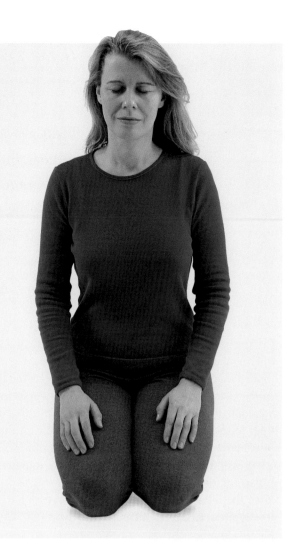

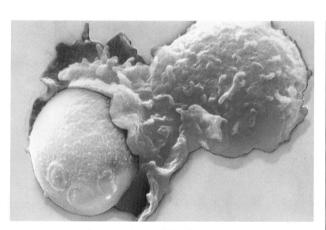

A lymphocyte – one of the immune system's protective cells – engulfs an alien yeast cell.

THE IMMUNE SYSTEM

The immune system is the body's reserve force in a marvelously ingenious system of defenses against the agents of disease. First-line defenses are devices such as eyelids, eyelashes, layers of skin, and the antiseptic fluid that bathes the eye. These stop almost anything – from insects and dust to bacteria – from entering the body. The last-line of defense is the immune response. This is the complex process by which clumps of proteins called antibodies are produced to attack and destroy any alien particle, such as a virus, which has managed to invade the body. Vaccination against diseases such as smallpox is an invasive way of maximizing the preventive powers of the immune system. Yoga searches for ways to strengthen and stimulate it, in the belief that its action is far more wide-ranging than just attacking and dealing with viruses. Breathing, meditation, and visualization are all techniques thought to stimulate the immune system.

Gentle stretching and breathing exercises used in yogic practice can help prevent a range of illnesses.

The Stress Factor

Stress symptoms can be relieved in one yoga session by stretching, relaxation, and breathing, and even by concentrating on performing a relaxing asana, such as the pose of tranquility. But the yoga approach is to get to the heart of the problem and to find a thorough, long-term solution. This involves searching for and experimenting with techniques which, in time, will eliminate its cause.

Yoga can relieve the symptoms and some of the causes of stress.

In the middle decades of the 20th century Hans Selye, a Hungarian studying medicine in Canada, noticed that patients with different diseases often have similar symptoms. He worked out that people suffer from what we now call stress. Selye identified two types of stress. The first, which derives from ordinary, predictable physical and mental action, he termed "eustress," meaning that it has no lasting impact and is part of daily life. The second type, which arises when the interplay of mind and body causes harmful psychophysical effects, he termed "distress." This is the type of stress that plays a role – often a pivotal one – in a wide range of health problems. It has taken some decades for Selye's theory to become accepted, but his distress, what he also called "unrelieved stress," is now accepted as the prolonged stress that can cause mental and physical damage. Today it is recognized that in economic terms alone, stress-related diseases cost every industrialized Western nation vast sums. The British government's Department of Health recently calculated the cost of stress to be about £5 billion ($8 billion) a year.

Many people turn to yoga to learn how to relieve what they feel must be the cause of their migraines, asthma, irritable bowel syndrome, ME, and other nervous and chronic ailments. Yoga responds by strengthening the body's own defense against illness, the immune system. Stimulating the electromagnetic system and the circulation of body fluids encourages the production of cells to attack harmful organisms. Yoga encourages a healthy diet and discourages indulgence in tobacco, alcohol, and coffee, which destroy the body's defenses. It also reduces the effects of stress, from chronic muscle rigidity to raised blood pressure.

FIRST AID FOR STRESS

Breathing can be used as a kind of psychic first aid when events get on top of you. To control the mental confusion, you must control your breathing.

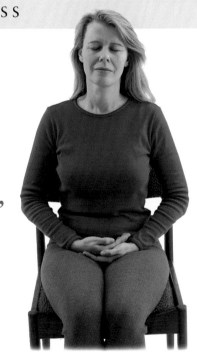

1 *Find a place you can be alone, stand or sit erect, and breathe slowly and rhythmically. To help your concentration, murmur the words on the right as you breathe.*

"Life is breath Breath is life"

2 *Mouth the words and breathe to the same rhythm and continue for as long as you feel you need to. If alarming thoughts intervene, gently push them away.*

3 *Focus your concentration on the mantra you are chanting and the timing of your breath until you feel more calm and better able to think more clearly.*

RELAXATION STRETCH

Regular reminders of the need to relax are good training for preventing a buildup of stress. This stretch helps you shake off the stresses of the day before you sleep. A short transition period when you relax and clear your mind of the day's events will help you sleep more deeply, so stressful events will be easier to deal with tomorrow. This exercise also makes a good starter in the morning.

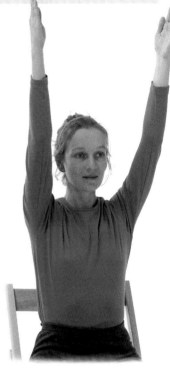

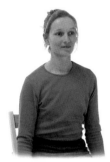

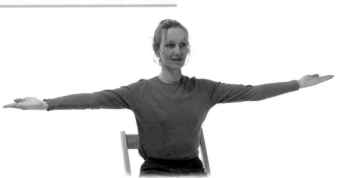

1 *Sit on the side of the bed or on a chair with your arms by your sides. Take a long out-breath.*

2 *Breathe in, stretching your arms right out to the sides and slowly stretching them up until they are straight above your head. Hold the stretch for some seconds.*

3 *Breathing out slowly, bring your arms down to your sides. Repeat the exercise once or twice. Then lie on your back in bed in the relaxation position until your breathing slows to a regular rhythm.*

RESTORING CALM

If you always seem to be in a state of stress, try visualizing one of these images. Practice at the same time every day if possible, paying attention to breathing. Begin by reminding yourself that nothing is so important it does not have another perspective.

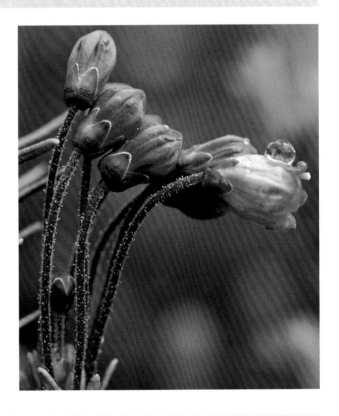

1 *Visualize a lovely scene with positive associations, such as a flower opening or the sun rising. Push aside all feelings of pressure, and fill your mind with the scene. Concentrate on it and the atmosphere of calm beauty it portrays. Do not allow negative thoughts to intervene.*

2 *Imagine yourself building a snowman on a cold winter day. Put all your energy, annoyance, and resentment into shoveling the snow. Spend all the time you need building the snowman, offloading all your stress onto him. When you outline his face, make him look happy, angry or sad, as you feel. Now, imagine the sun slowly melting the snowman, and all your resentments melting away.*

Flexible Body and Mind

Watch any accomplished yogi practicing asanas, and the elasticity of the muscular system is striking. The body seems capable of stretching into extraordinary postures. Students practicing to perfect difficult asanas are sometimes alarmed, therefore, to hear about articles that occasionally appear in physiotherapy journals suggesting that certain yoga postures damage the body by overstretching these muscles or straining those joints.

The difference between physiotherapy and yoga is that physiotherapy applies techniques to the body only, while yoga deals with body and mind. It starts from the premise that body and mind are inseparable, and its every approach addresses the interrelationship between the two.

Trying to force the muscles to bend the joints into extreme positions would, without doubt, cause damage. But gentle stretching aided by breathing and relaxation can, in time, persuade muscles and joints into positions that would normally be out of their range. In yoga, extreme positions are never adopted for the sake of it. Every yoga position has evolved because it benefits the body.

The flexibility of the human body is one of its great assets. It has its limitations – the head cannot be turned by 180° (although 90° or more is possible with practice) – and all bodies have their eccentricities, such as double-jointedness. It also has to be recog-

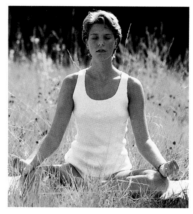

Yogis have studied nature and have produced asanas to stretch every part of the body and the mind.

nized that some parts of the body, such as the muscles that mobilize the lens of the eye, lose flexibility over time. Yoga helps students restore as much of the body's natural flexibilty as is possible, given their limitations. With dedication, discipline, and gentle persuasion, the final result is greatly improved maneuverability.

The natural integration of mind and body that is the aim of yoga requires equally that the flexibility of the mind be maintained. Yoga does this by exercising the power of visualization, and using it to find ways of controlling tension and restoring perspective in situations that threaten to overwhelm. The power of visualization enables people to understand that what they are seeing in many situations is a mere detail of a huge canvas, the shadow in the corner of a sunny landscape. Visualization enables the observer to stand back and appreciate the whole picture.

THE MENTAL COMPONENT OF EXERCISE

This simple exercise demonstrates the difference that the mind and the breathing make to the functioning of the neuromuscular system. There is a perceptible difference in sensation between raising the arm while breathing in and repeating the same movement while breathing out. It shows that the human being is an integrated unit and that to exercise one limb is to exercise the whole body and mind. Because of their mental component, the yoga asanas are not really exercises.

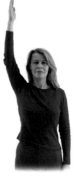

1 *Stand erect, breathe in, and raise one arm.*

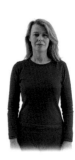

2 *Lower your arm, and breathe out.*

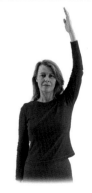

3 *This time, breathe out as you raise one arm.*

NATURAL ELASTICITY

Many yoga postures imitate the extraordinary elasticity of animals such as the cat. Children can imitate a cat with greater ease than many adults because their bodies still have their natural elasticity, and because they exercise constantly, practicing handstands and cartwheels. The flexible body needs maintenance, and you find it easier to maintain the younger you start. If you are an adult and you have not stretched your spine for years, it may hurt when you first try. You have to persist, quietly and calmly practicing for a minute or so a day, stopping when the pain begins. In time the minute will become two minutes and the pain, you will realize, was a temporary response to exercising a part of the body that needed to be used, not a sign that stretching the spine is an unnatural activity.

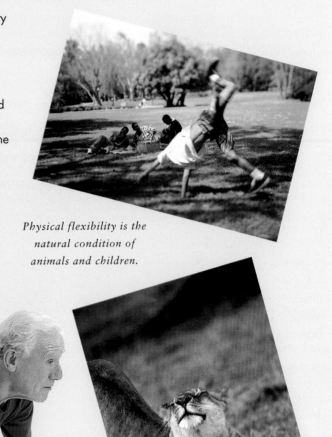

Physical flexibility is the natural condition of animals and children.

The cat pose

EXERCISING THE MIND

The mind becomes a tyrant if it is allowed to become rigid. Rigidity results from relinquishing control and allowing negative responses to dominate, so that everything seems terrible and other people seem unfriendly. Adults sometimes take up yoga because they feel instinctively that they have become too rigid. Yoga encourages people to relax into simplicity, to look outside and see that life is wonderful. Togetherness banishes rigidity and discussion encourages mental elasticity. When people talk to each other while practicing yoga, they find the asanas easier to achieve. And people with illnesses and disabilities find shared sessions and group discussions strengthen their ability to overcome their limitations.

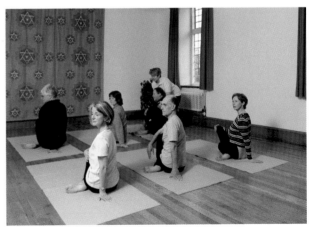

Communication between the teacher and the students is an important feature of any yoga class.

Peace through Reflection

···

*The holistic practice of yoga will bring inner peace and a deep sense of fulfillment.
Reading the ancient texts and the thoughts of wise people of modern times helps to
keep a perspective when everyday events threaten to take over. Even a busy life with
little time for reading and studying can benefit from recalling day by day the profound
statements of others. Here are some examples:*

*Wearing a particular type of dress
does not bring success; nor does talking
about one's yoga. Practicing alone
brings success: this undoubtedly
is the truth.*

SVATMARAMA, HATHAPRADIPIKA

*All rivers, whether they flow to the East
or to the West, have arisen from the sea
and will return to it again. Yet once
these rivers have merged with the sea
they no longer think, "I am this river,"
"I am that river." In the same way ... all
these creatures when they merge again
with Being, do not remember that they
originally arose from Being and wound
their individual ways through life.
Now that Being, which is the individual
essence of everything, the supreme
reality, the Self of all that exists,
THAT ART THOU.*

CHANDOGYA UPANISHAD

*The yogi sees himself in the heart of all
beings and sees all beings in his heart.*

BHAGAVAD GITA

Nothing can bring you peace but yourself.

RALPH WALDO EMERSON

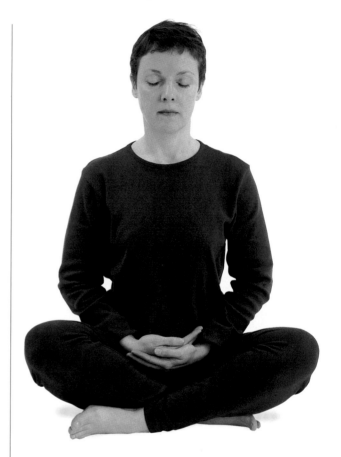

*Truth can be found by searching within,
never through debate or disputation.
It is just the same if for "Truth"
one reads "God."*

MOHANDAS KARAMCHAND
("MAHATMA") GANDHI

*The seed of mystery lies in muddy water.
How can I perceive this mystery?
Water becomes clear through stillness.
How can I become still?
By flowing with the stream.*

LAO TZU

Useful Addresses

THE YOGA FOR HEALTH FOUNDATION

Since its founding in 1976, the Yoga for Health Foundation has become an international organization. This listing gives contact addresses around the world.

UNITED KINGDOM AND IRISH REPUBLIC

The Yoga for Health Foundation
Ickwell Bury
Biggleswade
Bedfordshire
United Kingdom
SG18 9EF
Tel: 01767 627271
Fax: 01767 627 266

NORTHERN IRELAND

Northern Ireland Yoga Fellowship
Sharon Carmichael
8 Sinclair Park
Bangor
BT19 1PG

IRISH REPUBLIC

Phil Daly
117 Gaybrook Lawns
Malahide
Co. Dublin

ASIA

INDIA

Kaivalyadhama
Lonavla - 410 003
Maharashtra

HONG KONG

Martine Charpenet
East View, 12B
3 Cox's Road
Kowloon

NORTH AMERICA & THE CARIBBEAN

USA

Nancy Ford-Kohne
7918 Bolling Drive
Alexandria
Virginia 22308

CANADA

Margaret Gupta
2121 Galena Crescent
Oakville
Ontario L6H 4A9

Margaret McNair
1562 Southdown Road
Mississippi,
Ontario L5J 2Z4

BARBADOS

Diane Blades
Anbar
Cattlewash

AUSTRALIA & NEW ZEALAND

AUSTRALIA

Veronica Urquhart
PO Box 313
Montville
Queensland 4560

NEW ZEALAND

Terri Walsh
37 Te Henga Road
Henderson RD1
Auckland

AFRICA

SOUTH AFRICA

Stephanie Alexander
4 Barry Road
Pietermaritzburg 3021

GHANA

Sheridon Oliver
PO Box 65
International Trade Fair
Accra

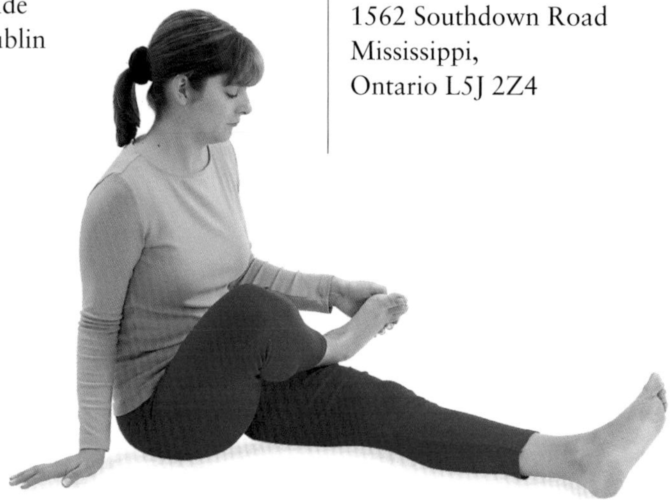

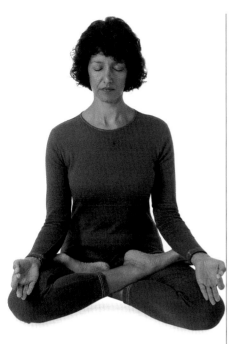

EUROPE

DENMARK

Pixi Lømberg-Holm
Bøgevonget 112
8310 Tranbjerg

LITHUANIA

Nikolai Scherbakov
Paberzes 14-100
Vilnius 2010

THE NETHERLANDS

Rik Verbeek
Reestraat 3
1016 DM
Amsterdam

PORTUGAL

Bea Fulcher
370 Vale Do Lobo
Almancil
Algarve

ROMANIA

Ekatarina Parus
Str. Progresului 8
Sc.3, Ap.23, Onesti 5450

SLOVAKIA

Sylvia Girling
Gymnázium a Sládkovica
Komenskémo 18
Banska Bystrica 97401

SPAIN

Jennifer Haberer
Apartamento Número 5
Cazorla
Jaen

RUSSIA

Dr Ludmila Kudaeva
bld 40/12
app 55
Novatorov's Street
117421 Moscow

MIDDLE EAST

EGYPT

*Scheherazade Moustapha
El Tarouti*
15 Abdel Khaler Sarwat
St Laurens
Alexandria

ISRAEL

Ilana Rathouse
Smuts 17
62009 Tel Aviv

OTHER ORGANIZATIONS:

Divine Life Society
Shivananddear
PT Tehri-Garhwal
Uttar Pradesh
India

Lonavla Yoga Institute
Lonavla - 410 401
India

British Wheel of Yoga
1 Hamilton Place
Boston Road
Stamford
Lincolnshire NG34 7ES
United Kingdom
Tel: 01529 306851

FOR INFORMATION ON
YOGA FOR MOTHERS AND
BABIES, CONTACT:

Yoga Therapy Centre
*Royal London
Homeopathic Hospital*
31-35 Great Ormond Street
London
United Kingdom
WC1 3HR
Tel: 0171 402 9200

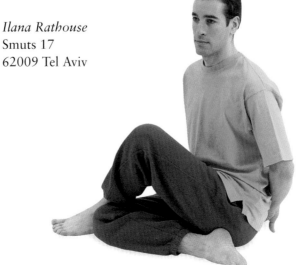

Further Reading

BOOKS BY THE AUTHOR:

Kent, Howard
Breathe Better Feel Better
APPLE PRESS 1997

Kent, Howard
Yoga for the Disabled
SUNRISE PUBLICATIONS 1985

Kent, Howard
The Complete Yoga Course
HEADLINE 1993

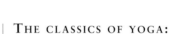

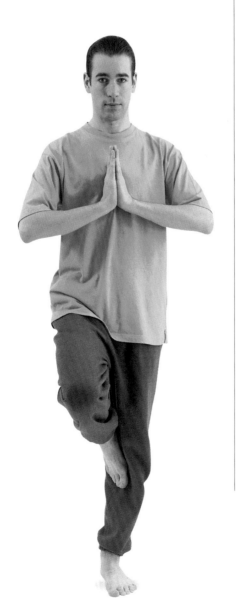

THE CLASSICS OF YOGA:

The Bhagavad Gita
translated by **Juan Mascaro**
PENGUIN BOOKS 1998

The Upanishads
translated by **Juan Mascaro**
PENGUIN BOOKS 1998

The Upanishads
translated by **S. Nikhilananda**
RAMAKRISHNA-VIVEKANANDA CENTER,
NEW YORK 1993

Wisdom of the Upanishads
NEW AGE PUBLICATIONS 1995

The Yoga Sutras of Patañjali
New Translation and Commentary: "Enlightenment"
SFA PUBLICATIONS 1995

The Yoga Sutras of Patañjali
ASIAN HUMANITIES PRESS, USA 1993

Iyengar, B.K.S.
Light on The Yoga Sutras of Patañjali
AQUARIAN PRESS 1998

Yogananda Metaphysical Meditations
SELF-REALIZATION FELLOWSHIP, USA 1998

GENERAL:

Fontana, David
A Meditator's Handbook, A Comprehensive Guide to Eastern and Western Meditation Techniques
ELEMENT BOOKS 1998

Hittleman, Richard
Yoga: A 28-Day Exercise Plan
BANTAM, USA 1998

Iyengar, B.K.S.
Light on Yoga
AQUARIAN PRESS 1991; SCHOCKEN,
NEW YORK, USA 1996

Iyengar, B.K.S.
Tree of Yoga
AQUARIAN PRESS 1998

Sturgess, Stephen
The Yoga Book
ELEMENT BOOKS 1997

Prabhavananda, Swami
Spiritual Heritage of India
VEDANTA PUBLICATIONS, USA 1993

Vishnudevananda, Swami
The Complete Illustrated Book of Yoga
YES INTERNATIONAL, USA 1996

Yogananda, Paramahansa
Autobiography of a Yogi
RIDER 1991

Yogananda, Mata
Self-Realization through Meditation
DAOSEVA PRESS 1994

SPECIALIST:

Mainland, Pauline
A Yoga Parade of Animals,
A First Fun Picture Book on Yoga
ELEMENT 1998

Balaskas, Janet
Preparing for Birth with Yoga
ELEMENT 1994

Olkin, Silvia Klein
Positive Pregnancy Fitness, A Guide to
a More Comfortable Pregnancy and Easier Birth
Through Exercise and Relaxation
AVERY PUBLICATIONS, USA 1996

Weller, Stella
Yoga Therapy: Safe Natural Methods to Promote
Healing and Restore Health and Well-Being
THORSONS 1998

Weller, Stella
Yoga Back Book
THORSONS 1998

Friedman, Miriam and Hankee, Janice
Yoga at Work
ELEMENT 1996

Agombar, Fiona
Beat Fatigue with Yoga
ELEMENT 1999

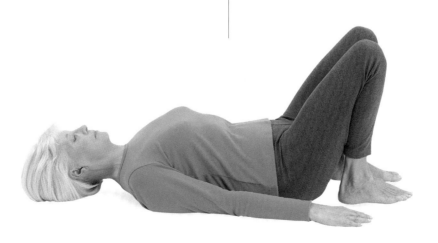

Glossary

A

ahimsa
living one's life without violence in thought, word, or deed. Ahimsa is the first of the five rules of conduct called yamas (q.v.)

ananda
bliss

asana *(ah-sna)*
yoga posture or position

ashram
a place of holy study

asteya
never taking anything that belongs to another. Asteya is the second of the five rules of conduct called yamas (q.v.)

atman
consciousness

B

bhakti
devotion or adoration

bandhas
movements that involve blocking the out-breath temporarily

brahmacharya
the control of lust

brahman
Hindu priest; also an Indian caste

C

chakra
wheel of energy; a vortex of energy in the body

ch'i or ji
the Chinese word for life force

citta
mental activity

D

dharana
concentration

dhyana
contemplation

E

electro-magnetic energy
the flow of electrically charged chemical particles that circulates around the body in the blood and tissue fluid

G

glottis
a narrow opening between the vocal cords

gunas
the three threads that intertwine with the physical world and the universal consciousness to produce life. *See also sattva; rajas; tamas*

H

hatha yoga
a way of attaining yoga through practicing asanas, breathing, and cleansing processes, which evolved about 1,000 years ago

I

immune system
the body's complex system of defences against invasion by agents of disease

J

jnana
knowledge or wisdom. Jnana yoga is the yoga of the intellect

K

karma
work or destiny. Karma yoga is the yoga of selfless action.

M

mantra
literally "an instrument of thought" – words or sounds used as a focus for concentration

meridian
the Chinese word used in acupuncture for the pathways along which energy (ch'i or qi) flows around the body. The Sanskrit word, used in yoga, is nadi (q.v.)

mudras
movements that involve imitating natural actions of the body

N

nada
a ringing sound

nadis
the channels or meridians along with energy flows around the body

niyamas
the principles governing the way we relate to ourselves

O

om
the primal sound of the universe, often used as a mantra

P

prakriti
the physical universe

prana
life energy

pranayamas
energy-expanding techniques

pratyahara
the control of the senses

purakha
inspiration or breathing in

purusha
universal consciousness

R

raja
royal or ruler

rajas
the second of the gunas (q.v.): the force of energy

rechakh
expiration or breathing out

S

samadhi
meditation; enlightenment

samkya
exact knowledge

santosha
equanimity

sattva
the first of the gunas (q.v.): the pure life force

satya
always speaking the truth. Satya is the fourth of the five rules of conduct called yamas (q.v.)

shauca
inner and outer purity. Shauca is the first of the five rules of conduct called niyamas (q.v.)

shavasana
relaxation; the corpse position

swami
holy man

T

tamas
the third of the gunas (q.v.), the force of inertia

tapas
the ability to rise above objects of desire. Tapas is the second of the five rules of conduct called niyamas (q.v.)

Y

yamas
principles governing the way to relate to other people

yoga
oneness

POSITIONS, MOVEMENTS, AND TECHNIQUES

ardha-matsyendrasana
half twist

bhastrika
bellows breath

bhoomi sparsh mudra
touching the earth

bhramari
black bee

bhujangasana
cobra

chakrasana
the wheel

dhanurasana
bow

halasana
plow

kapalabhati
shining head breath

konasana
triangle

kumbhaka
restraining or holding the breath
matsyasana
fish

matsyendranana
twist

nadi shuddan
alternate nostril breath

namaste
prayer position

naukasana
canoe

padhastasana
stretch

padmasana
lotus

parvatasana
mountain

pashchimottasana
forward bend

shalabhasana
locust

sharvangasana
shoulder stand

shavasana
the corpse; relaxation

simbhasana
lion

sitkari
cooling breath

suryanamaskar
salute to the sun

trikonasana
triangle

vajrasana
sitting on the heels

vrikshasana
tree

Index

Acknowledgments

The Publishers are grateful to the following for permission to reproduce copyright material:

AKG: pp. 14T, 16B, 21BR, 131C, 139T
Bridgeman Art Library: pp. 14B (Victoria & Albert Museum, London), 16T (British Museum), 136BR (Brooklyn Museum, New York), 138T (Victoria & Albert Museum, London), 138B (British Library)
European Space Agency: p. 30T
Derek Heape: p. 118
Hulton Getty: pp. 17T, 136BL
Michael Holford: p. 134T
Hutchison Library: pp. 18, 20BR, 32T
Image Bank: pp. 28, 122B
Rex Features: pp. 10BL, 17BR
Science Photo Library: pp. 25CR, 25CL, 25BR, 25BL, 47BL, 140B, 175BL
Stock Market: pp. 10 BR, 42, 130BR
Tony Stone Images: pp. 15, 20BC, 21BC, 25TR, 25 TL, 26, 27BL, 29B, 31T, 31B, 32B, 46T, 48T, 62BL, 98T, 110BL, 110BR, 122T, 124, 125TL, 126T, 127BR, 134BL, 134BR, 136T, 140T, 141TR, 144BR, 145T, 145C, 145B, 147T, 147TC, 147BC, 147B, 148BR, 151CR, 151BR, 170T, 174B, 177BR, 178T, 179TR, 179CR, 181
Trip: pp. 17BL, 130BL, 148BL

Special thanks to Ann Davenport, Natalie Davenport, Philip Lloyd Davenport, Elizabeth Longland, Shirley Mindell, Kathryn Relton, Howard Smith, Cath Stoup, Helen Webb, Rosie and William Wright, and The Yoga for Health Foundation for help with photography.

Special thanks to Brian at the Rivendell Retreat Centre, Chillies Lane, High Hurstwood, East Sussex for making and supplying the meditation beads.

Howard Kent wishes to express his warm appreciation for the invaluable assistance given by Helen Varley in the preparation of this book.

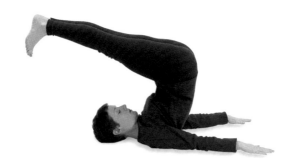